Nuclear Magnetic Resonance Spectroscopy

NMR
An Introduction to Proton

Nuclear Magnetic Resonance Spectroscopy

ADDISON AULT
Cornell College
Mt. Vernon, Iowa

GERALD O. DUDEK
Harvard University
Cambridge, Massachusetts

HOLDEN-DAY, INC,. San Francisco

Düsseldorf   Johannesburg   London   Mexico
Panama   Sao Paulo   Singapore   Sydney

NMR
An Introduction To Proton
Nuclear Magnetic Resonance Spectroscopy

Copyright © 1976 by Holden-Day, Inc.
500 Sansome Street, San Francisco, California 94111

Library of Congress Catalog Card Number: 75-26286
ISBN: 0-8162-0331-8

Printed in the United States of America

234567890   CO   09876

Preface

The purpose of this book is to provide an introduction to the techniques and the theory of NMR spectroscopy that will make it possible for the student reader to obtain and interpret the proton NMR spectrum of a simple unknown organic compound.

Although most introductory organic texts present a discussion of NMR spectroscopy, the treatment is usually rather brief. Also, while many organic laboratory manuals mention NMR spectroscopy, few discuss the interpretation of spectra, and almost none tell how to prepare the sample or how to obtain a spectrum. Now that NMR has become such an important part of organic chemistry and proton NMR spectrometers have become widely available, we believe that many teachers and students will want to give more emphasis to the theory and practice of NMR spectrometry. This short introductory book is designed to facilitate a more thorough treatment. The first chapters introduce the NMR effect and describe the three main features of a proton NMR spectrum: the chemical shift differences, the integral, and the spin-spin splitting patterns. Next, first-order splitting patterns are discussed and illustrated, and then distorted first-order and complex splitting patterns are described. Magnetic equivalence is correctly defined. Chapter 7 presents the interpretation of the proton NMR spectra of a number of compounds of known structure and tells how to approach the interpretation of the spectra of unknown compounds. Two chapters then describe practical aspects of preparing the sample and obtaining the spectrum, and a final chapter mentions a few of the other applications and techniques of NMR spectrometry. Many problems are presented at the ends of the chapters.

ADDISON AULT
Mt. Vernon, Iowa

GERALD O. DUDEK
Cambridge, Massachusetts

Contents

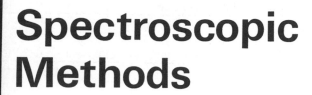

Spectroscopic Methods

Spectroscopic methods are concerned with the measurement of the extent to which electromagnetic radiation (radiant energy) is absorbed or emitted by samples of materials. The degree of absorption or emission of electromagnetic radiation varies with its wavelength, and the record of the extent of absorption or emission as a function of wavelength is called the absorption or emission spectrum.

Spectroscopic methods may be classified either according to the portion of the electromagnetic spectrum involved or according to the atomic or molecular mechanism considered to be responsible for the absorption of the radiant energy. For example, the terms ultraviolet-visible spectroscopy and electronic spectroscopy are often used interchangeably since the mechanism of energy absorption in this part of the electromagnetic spectrum usually involves the excitation of an electron from a lower electronic energy level to a higher one. Similarly, infrared spectroscopy is often called vibrational spectroscopy or vibrational-rotational spectroscopy, and microwave spectroscopy may be called rotational spectroscopy. Figure 1-1 shows the relationships between the energy, frequency, and wavelength of electromagnetic radiation. It also indicates some of the regions of the electromagnetic spectrum.

From Figure 1-1 you can see that nuclear magnetic resonance (NMR) spectroscopy involves the absorption of electromagnetic radiation in the radiofrequency portion of the spectrum and that the radiant energy involved is very slight. Chapter 2 describes the process by which the radiant energy in this part of the electromagnetic spectrum is absorbed.

One reason spectroscopic methods are of use to the chemist is that if the mechanism of energy absorption is known in terms of molecular structure, the spectra of molecules of unknown structure can then be interpreted in terms of features of molecular structure that must be either present or absent.

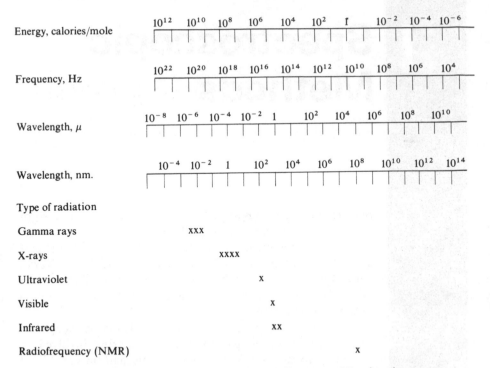

Figure 1-1   The Electromagnetic Spectrum: Energy, Frequency, Wavelength.

Before the development of NMR spectroscopy, infrared spectroscopy was most useful in this respect, since the presence or absence of absorption at certain wavelengths could be correlated with the presence or absence of certain functional groups or combinations of atoms. At present, NMR spectroscopy is almost as widely and extensively used, the reason being that features of the NMR spectrum can be interpreted in great detail (1) in terms of the presence or absence of certain magnetic nuclei in different functional groups and (2) in terms of the structural and geometric relationships among the magnetic nuclei.

NMR techniques are also extensively used in studying chemical and conformational equilibria and rates and mechanisms of chemical reactions.

2 Basis of the Nuclear Magnetic Resonance Effect

2.1 MAGNETIC PROPERTIES OF ATOMIC NUCLEI

Some atomic nuclei—e.g., the most abundant isotopes of carbon (^{12}C) and oxygen (^{16}O)—have no magnetic properties. Others—such as the most abundant isotopes of hydrogen (^{1}H; the proton), fluorine (^{19}F), and phosphorous (^{31}P)—appear to behave as magnets. When placed in a magnetic field they have a preferred (lowest energy) orientation, just like a compass needle in the earth's magnetic field.

Work must be done on the magnet (i.e., energy must be added to the system) in order to move the magnet to a less preferred, higher energy orientation. Although a compass needle can be made to assume practically any orientation in relation to the earth's magnetic field, in the three magnetically active nuclei mentioned—^{1}H, ^{19}F, and ^{31}P—only two orientations are possible—one of lower energy ("with" the external magnetic field) and one of higher energy ("against" it). These three nuclei possess *magnetic dipoles*. The difference in energy of the two orientations, ΔE, is proportional to the strength of the magnetic field experienced by the nucleus, $H_{at\ nucleus}$:

$$(2\text{-}1) \qquad \Delta E \propto H_{at\ nucleus}$$

The greater the magnetic field, the greater the energy difference of the nucleus in the two states.

When a large number of the nuclei of a particular magnetically active isotope in a magnetic field reaches thermal equilibrium, more nuclei will be in a lower energy state than in an upper energy state. The relative numbers in the two states will correspond to the Boltzman distribution:

$$(2\text{-}2) \qquad \frac{\text{number in upper state}}{\text{number in lower state}} = e^{-\Delta E/RT}$$

For the ordinary magnetic fields that are experimentally available, ΔE is so small compared (at room temperature) to RT there will be almost as many nuclei in the upper state as in the lower state. For protons, for example, where $H_{at\ nucleus} = 14{,}092$ gauss in a NMR spectrometer, $\Delta E = 0.0057$ calories/mole. Since at room temperature, $RT = 592$ calories/mole, $\Delta E/RT = 1 \times 10^{-5}$, and therefore out of 2,000,010 nuclei, 1,000,000 would be in the upper state and 1,000,010 in the lower. This is in distinct contrast with electronic energy levels where the difference between energy levels ΔE, is so large that at room temperature practically every molecule is in its ground electronic state, and with vibrational energy levels where a population of a few percent in the first excited state is relatively high.

Table 2-1 summarizes the magnetic properties of some atomic nuclei.

Table 2-1   Magnetic Properties of Selected Atomic Nuclei

Isotope	NMR frequency for a 14,092 gauss field, MHz	Natural abundance, %	Relative sensitivity	Magnetic moment, μ	Spin quantum number, I
^1H	60.000	99.9844	1.000	2.79270	1/2
^2H	9.210	0.0156	0.009	0.85738	1
^{12}C		98.892			0
^{13}C	15.086	1.108	0.016	0.70220	1/2
^{14}N	4.335	99.635	0.001	0.40358	1
^{15}N	6.081	0.365	0.001	−0.28304	1/2
^{16}O		99.76			0
^{17}O	8.134	0.037	0.029	−1.8930	5/2
^{19}F	56.447	100	0.834	2.6273	1/2
^{31}P	24.290	100	0.066	1.1305	1/2

2.2 MECHANISM OF ENERGY ABSORPTION

As in ultraviolet and infrared spectroscopy, transitions or jumps between two energy states can occur if the nuclei are irradiated with electromagnetic radiation for which the energy (Planck's constant times the frequency) exactly equals the difference in energy of the two states:

$$(2\text{-}3) \qquad\qquad h v = \Delta E$$

Since according to Equation 2-1 the difference in energy of the two levels depends upon the magnetic field experienced by the nuclei, the frequency of the electromagnetic radiation that will cause transitions between the two levels depends upon the strength of the magnetic field:

$$(2\text{-}4) \qquad\qquad h v \propto H_{at\ nucleus}$$

For protons experiencing a field at the nucleus of 14,092 gauss, the frequency of electromagnetic radiation required is 60 megahertz (60 MHz = 60 megacycles/

second). This is in the radiofrequency part of the electromagnetic spectrum, and radiation of this type is often referred to as an *rf field*.

Since there are a few more nuclei in the lower state than in the upper, and since the probability of a downward transition for a nucleus in the upper level is equal to the probability of an upward transition for a nucleus in the lower level, then irradiation of the nuclei in the magnetic field with an rf field of the correct frequency will result in a net absorption of energy by the nuclei since there will be a few more upward transitions than downward transitions. In the cases of infrared and ultraviolet spectroscopy, the possibility of downward transitions or jumps is usually ignored since few molecules are in any state but the ground state. A net excess of downward transitions is the basis for laser action.

Figure 2-1 shows a block diagram for a "double coil" NMR spectrometer. The transmitter coil introduces the rf field, and the coil surrounding the sample

Figure 2-1   Block Diagram of a Double Coil NMR Spectrometer.

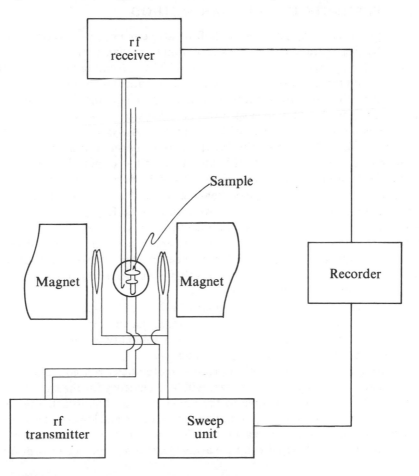

detects the extent of energy absorption by the sample. The sweep coil permits variation of the magnetic field experienced by the sample.

The fact that for any one type of nucleus the transition probability is essentially independent of the structural environment of the nuclei, means that a determination of the relative intensity of two different absorptions is a measure of the relative number of the nuclei responsible for the different absorptions. Again, this is in contrast to infrared and ultraviolet spectroscopy, where the intrinsic strength of absorption bands may differ greatly as, for example, carbon-oxygen double bonds absorb much more strongly in the infrared than do carbon-carbon double bonds. For this reason, the relative strengths of the carbonyl absorption and the carbon-carbon double bond absorption could not be taken as a measure of the relative amounts of a ketone and an alkene in a mixture. However, the relative amounts of components of mixtures may be determined by measuring the relative strengths of their NMR absorption bands; this is one important application of NMR spectroscopy.

2.3 SENSITIVITY OF THE NMR METHOD

Although it is possible under the most favorable circumstances to obtain useful proton NMR spectra from solutions containing less than 1 milligram of sample, most routine spectra will involve the use of 25 to 50 milligrams of sample in about $\frac{1}{2}$ milliliter of solvent. This sample concentration is two to five times greater than that used for a routine infrared spectrum, and 100 to 1000 times greater than that for ultraviolet spectroscopy. Thus you can see that NMR spectroscopy is not a particularly sensitive method of analysis.

While the sensitivity of the NMR method depends primarily upon the strength of the nuclear magnet, it is also affected by certain experimental variables. The most important of these is the strength of the external magnetic field, H_{ext}, which provides the magnetic field experienced by the nucleus, $H_{at\ nucleus}$. Since ΔE in Equation 2-2 increases with increasing $H_{at\ nucleus}$, the use of a larger magnetic field in the NMR experiment will result in a larger excess of nuclei in the lower state relative to the upper state and hence a greater net absorption of energy. Although most proton NMR spectrometers employ a magnetic field of 14,092 gauss, there exist spectrometers that use superconducting magnets with a field strength of more than 50,000 gauss.

It should be apparent from Equation 2-2 that the excess of nuclei in the lower state could also be increased by performing the experiment at a lower temperature. However, because of decreasing solubility at lower temperatures and other factors, this approach is of limited value.

During the energy absorption process, more nuclei will go from the lower energy state to the upper, and so there will be a tendency for the small excess of nuclei in the lower state relative to the upper state to diminish. If this process approaches completion (if the populations of the upper and lower stated approach equality—if *saturation* takes place), there can no longer be a net absorption of energy and the NMR signal will fade away. Therefore if energy absorption by a set of magnetic nuclei is to be maintained more than momentarily, there must be a way for the original small excess of nuclei in the lower state to be restored. That is, there must exist *relaxation* processes by which nuclei in the upper state can lose energy. The rates of relaxation are different for different kinds of nuclei, some having a half-time of many seconds. The rates can also vary for the same kind of nucleus in different structural environments. If the rate of relaxation is low (if the relaxation time is long), this will limit the amount of energy that can be absorbed and thus reduce the sensitivity. It is possible to measure relaxation times and thereby obtain information that can provide valuable clues to molecular structure. This technique is especially useful in ^{13}C NMR studies. Experimental variables that affect the rates of saturation and relaxation will be discussed in Chapter 9.

In both infrared and ultraviolet spectroscopy, the excess of molecules in the lower state is so large and the rates of relaxation so great that saturation is never a problem. The momentary burst of energy from a laser is the result of a stimulated simultaneous relaxation of the net excess of molecules or atoms in an excited state.

3 Features of the Nuclear Magnetic Resonance Spectrum

3.1 THE CHEMICAL SHIFT

If a substance containing magnetically active nuclei (^{1}H, ^{19}F, ^{31}P, etc.) is placed in a magnetic field, energy will be absorbed when the frequency of the radiation of an rf field corresponds to the difference between energy levels (Equation 2-3). For any given magnetic field strength, the frequency of the rf field required will be quite different for each different kind of magnetically active nucleus, as indicated in Table 2-1. Conversely, for an rf field of a particular frequency, the magnetic field strength required for energy absorption (resonance) of different kinds of magnetically active nuclei will also be quite different. These differences are so large that the NMR spectrum of any one type of magnetically active nucleus can be recorded without overlap from any other.

However, the great usefulness of the NMR method for the chemist derives from the fact that for any particular type of magnetic nucleus the strength of the external magnetic field, H_{ext}, required to provide a field at the nucleus, $H_{at\ nucleus}$, of exactly the right size will vary slightly with the structural environment of the nucleus. This small variation is called the *chemical shift*. The phenomenon of the chemical shift will be illustrated with reference to proton NMR spectroscopy but the idea applies in a similar way to the NMR spectroscopy of any other magnetically active nucleus.

If a sample* of a substance containing protons is placed in a magnetic field and irradiated by a 60 MHz rf field, energy will be absorbed due to the NMR effect if the magnetic field experienced by some of the protons in the sample is equal to

---

* As explained in Section 8.1, the sample is usually a pure liquid or a solution.

14,092 gauss. To a first approximation, the field at the nucleus, $H_{at\ nucleus}$, equals that of the external magnetic field, H_{ext}, minus a very small amount, $H_{shielding}$, by which the external field is diminished by the effect of the electrons in the environment of the proton:

$$H_{at\ nucleus} = H_{ext} - H_{shielding}$$

The effect of the electrons in the environment of the protons is always to react to create a small magnetic field that opposes the external or applied field and thus make the field at the nucleus smaller than the external field; the electrons "shield" the nucleus. It happens that the electronic environments of protons in various functional groups are sufficiently different that slightly different values of H_{ext} are required to make $H_{at\ nucleus}$ equal to 14,092 gauss for protons in different functional groups. Thus if the sample in the magnetic field H_{ext} is irradiated with a constant rf field of exactly 60 MHz and H_{ext} is slowly increased, energy will be absorbed by the sample each time $H_{at\ nucleus}$ (which equals $H_{ext} - H_{shielding}$) becomes equal to 14,092 gauss. Thus a graph of energy absorption versus H_{ext} is the NMR spectrum. The NMR spectrum of benzene would

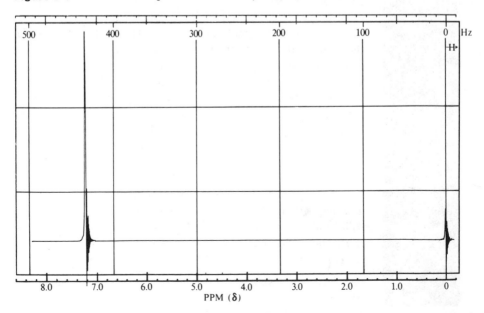

benzene

Figure 3-1   Proton NMR Spectrum of Benzene; CCl_4 Solution.

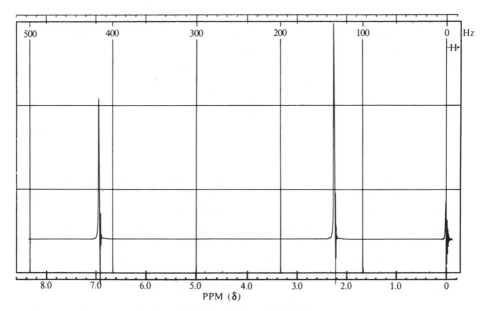

Figure 3-2   Proton NMR Spectrum of *p*-Xylene; CCl₄ Solution.

show only a single instance of energy absorption—a single resonance (Figure 3-1)—whereas the spectrum of *p*-xylene would show two resonances, one for the methyl protons, and one for the ring protons (Figure 3-2). This difference in the

para-xylene

external field, H_{ext}, required for the resonance of different protons is called the *difference in chemical shift*, $\Delta\delta$. It is important to remember that shielding and therefore chemical shift differences are proportional to the strength of H_{ext}.

Since it is difficult to determine the absolute value of H_{ext} to the required accuracy of about 1 part in 100,000,000, resonances are described by their displacement from the resonance of a reference substance that is added to the sample whose NMR spectrum is being determined. For protons, a commonly used reference substance is tetramethylsilane (TMS). A magnetic field unit of

tetramethylsilane (TMS)

convenient size to describe this small displacement is one millionth of the magnitude of the external field, 1 part per million, (1 ppm). This **fractional** type of unit has the advantage of being independent of the magnitude of H_{ext} even though shielding depends upon the strength of the external field. Thus it is possible to directly compare chemical shift data obtained from instruments employing external fields (and therefore rf fields) of different magnitude. For example, instrument A uses an external field of 14,092 gauss and instrument B uses one twice as great. Although the shielding determined by instrument B will be twice that determined by instrument A, it will be the same **fraction** of the external magnetic field in each case.

One set of units, δ units, sets the position of the resonance of the highly shielded TMS protons at zero and gives less shielded protons more positive values. Since some felt that less shielding ought to be associated with a smaller number, an alternative set of units, τ units, was proposed: $\tau = 10 - \delta$. On this scale, the resonance of the standard TMS, has the value 10 and less shielded protons have smaller, positive values down to zero. Both sets of units are used, but the size of the unit is the same in both cases—1 ppm of the external field. (Although H_{ext} does vary in the course of the experiment, its total variation is about 10 ppm (0.001 percent) and may be ignored for the purpose of determining the size of the unit of chemical shift.)

Although the NMR experiment as just described involves a constant value for the frequency of rf radiation and a variable external magnetic field, H_{ext}, the experiment may be done the other way around. In this case H_{ext} is held constant and the frequency of the rf field is varied so that groups of nuclei experiencing different total fields at the nucleus—which equal $H_{ext} - H_{shielding}$—will be subjected in turn to an rf field of the correct frequency to result in energy absorption. Thus the NMR spectrum will be a record of energy absorption versus frequency of electromagnetic radiation, in analogy with infrared and ultraviolet spectroscopy. The resulting record of energy absorption versus rf field frequency (H_{ext} constant) will look exactly like the record of energy absorption versus H_{ext} (rf field constant). From this second way of doing the experiment, you can see that chemical shifts could be expressed as parts per million of the frequency of the rf field; 1 ppm of 60 MHz is 60 Hz (cycles per second). Frequency units like this will be useful in comparing the magnitude of chemical shift differences, $\Delta\delta$, with coupling constants, J, which are expressed in cycles per second. Figure 3-3 shows the relationships between the three sets of chemical shift units for protons.

Now that the NMR spectra of a great many compounds of known structure have been determined, it has become apparent that the position of resonance of a magnetically active nucleus relative to a reference standard for that nucleus varies in a regular way that depends upon the structural environment of the nucleus. For example, the protons of a $-CH_3$ group bonded to a saturated carbon atom have a chemical shift of about 0.9 to 1.1δ, and the protons of a $-CH_3$ group bonded to oxygen have a chemical shift of about 3.2 to 3.4δ. The overall range of proton chemical shifts is about 20 ppm.

Increasing H_{ext} →
Increasing frequency ←
Increasing shielding →

11	10	9	8	7	6	5	4	3	2	1	0	−1	δ
−1	0	1	2	3	4	5	6	7	8	9	10	11	τ
330	300	270	240	210	180	150	120	90	60	30	0	−30	Hz[a]
660	600	540	480	420	360	300	240	180	120	60	0	−60	Hz[b]
1100	1000	900	800	700	600	500	400	300	200	100	0	−100	Hz[c]

[a]30 MHz instrument
[b]60 MHz instrument
[c]100 MHz instrument

↑
Position of TMS resonance

Figure 3-3   Units of Chemical Shift

A good example of how it is possible in a favorable case to calculate an expected proton chemical shift is found with compounds of the type $X-CH_2-Y$. Table 3-1 gives "effective shielding constants" for various X and Y that when

Table 3-1   Effective Shielding Constants for Compounds of the Type $X-CH_2-Y$

X or Y	Effective shielding constant
$-CH_3$	0.47
$-C\!=\!C$	1.32
$\overset{\displaystyle O}{\overset{\|}{-C-O-}}$	1.55
$\overset{\displaystyle O}{\overset{\|}{-C-R}}$	1.70
$-I$	1.82
$-\phi$	1.85
$-Br$	2.33
$-OR$	2.36
$-Cl$	2.53
$-OH$	2.56
$-O-\overset{\displaystyle O}{\overset{\|}{C}}-$	3.23
$-O-\phi$	3.23

The chemical shift of the $-CH_2-$ protons in compounds of the type $X-CH_2-Y$ may be estimated by adding the "effective shielding constants" for X and Y to 0.23. The sum will give the expected chemical shift of the $-CH_2-$ protons in δ units.

added to 0.23, will give the expected chemical shift for the methylene protons in δ units. For example, benzyl bromide ($\phi-CH_2-Br$) should show a peak for the methylene protons at $0.23 + 1.85 + 2.33 = 4.41\delta$; the observed value is 4.3δ. It is apparent from Table 3-1 that the greater the electron-withdrawing ability of the substituent, the less the shielding. This is consistent with the notion that shielding is due to the electron density around the magnetically active nucleus. (The dependence of chemical shift values upon molecular structure will be described in greater detail for protons in Section 7.1.)

3.2 THE INTEGRAL

Since the degree to which energy is absorbed by any particular type of magnetically active nucleus is independent of its structural environment, the total area, or integral, of an absorption peak is proportional to the number of nuclei responsible for the absorption. The area is normally determined electronically with the NMR spectrometer in a separate operation after obtaining the absorption spectrum. The vertical displacement of the second trace is proportional to the area under the corresponding peak. Figure 3-4 shows the NMR spectrum of p-xylene and its integral. The area of the resonance of the ring protons is seen to be two-thirds that of the methyl protons. The integral thus gives information about the relative number of nuclei for which resonance occurs at different chemical shifts.

In the case of the NMR spectrum of a pure compound, it may be possible to estimate the total number of magnetically active nuclei of a particular type in a molecule from the integral. For example, if in a proton NMR spectrum the

Figure 3-4   Proton NMR Spectrum and Integral of p-Xylene; CCl_4 Solution.

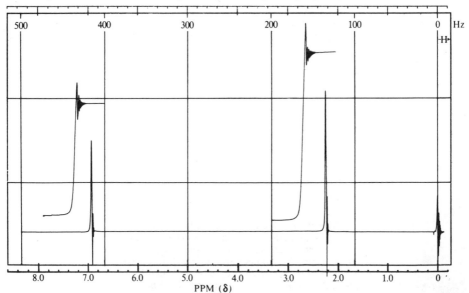

integral of the entire spectrum is four times the integral of a resonance which you believe corresponds to a methyl group, the total number of protons must be four times the number in a methyl group, or twelve.

If the NMR spectrum is that of a mixture, it may be possible to estimate the composition of the mixture from the NMR spectrum. To choose an easy example, suppose we have a mixture of two substances each of which contains a methyl group and the methyl resonances appear at different chemical shifts. The ratio of the integrals of the peaks for the two methyl groups in the proton NMR spectrum will equal the molecular or molar ratio of the two components. With care this ratio can be determined to ± 1 percent.

3.3   THE SPLITTING PATTERN

We have now seen that protons in different molecular environments can be expected to give resonances at different chemical shifts. We have also seen that the integral of each resonance is proportional to the number of protons responsible for each resonance. We will see next that there is an additional feature of the NMR spectrum that can give information as to the structural and geometrical relationships between the various magnetically active nuclei in a molecule.

The proton NMR spectrum of 1,1,2,2-tetrachloroethane is shown in Figure

$$
\begin{array}{cc}
\text{Cl} & \text{Cl} \\
| & | \\
\text{H--C--C-} & \text{II} \\
| & | \\
\text{Cl} & \text{Cl}
\end{array}
$$

1,1,2,2-tetrachloroethane

3-5. The fact that the spectrum consists of only one resonance (a *singlet*) is consistent with our understanding that in this molecule the two protons experience the same molecular environment.

Figure 3-6 shows the proton NMR spectrum of 1,1-dibromo-2,2-dichloroethane. From what has been said so far, one would expect the proton NMR

$$
\begin{array}{cc}
\text{Br} & \text{Cl} \\
| & | \\
\text{H}_A\text{--C--C--H}_x \\
| & | \\
\text{Br} & \text{Cl}
\end{array}
$$

1,1-dibromo-2,2-dichloroethane

spectrum of this compound to consist of two singlets, one for each of the structurally different protons. The spectrum actually shows four lines, two for each proton. The resonance of each proton has been split into a doublet by its single neighbor at a different chemical shift.

This example of *splitting* can be explained by a very simple model. As stated in Section 2.1, a particular proton in a magnetic field has an almost equal chance of being in either the lower or higher energy spin state, of being oriented either with or against the external magnetic field. Therefore according to this model, you can estimate that one-half the molecules will have the X proton

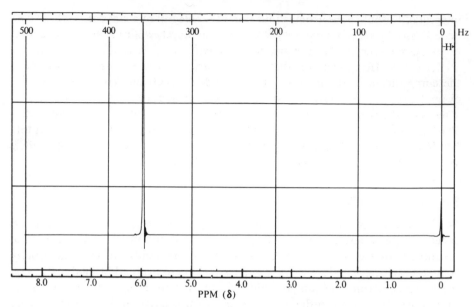

Figure 3-5 Proton NMR Spectrum of 1,1,2,2-Tetrachloroethane; CDCl₃ Solution.

oriented with H_{ext}, or ↑, and one-half the molecules will have the X proton oriented against H_{ext}, or ↓. The effect of having the X proton oriented with the external field will be to bring the A proton of those molecules into resonance at

Figure 3-6 1,1-Dibromo-2,2-dichloroethane. (Since an authentic spectrum of 1,1-dibromo-2,2-dichloroethane was not available, this is simulated spectrum.)

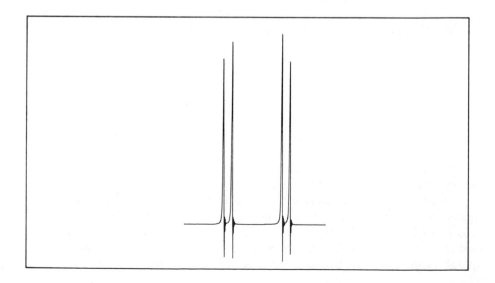

a slightly lower value of H_{ext}. This is because the X proton oriented with the field will augment H_{ext} for its neighbor H_A. This effect of the neighboring proton may be expressed by Equation 3-1, where $H_{coupling}$ is positive. Thus the H_A

(3-1) $$H_{at\,nucleus} = H_{ext} - H_{shielding} + H_{coupling}$$

resonance for half the molecules will occur at slightly lower field (smaller H_{ext}) than would be expected in the absence of this coupling. In the other half of the molecules the X protons are oriented against H_{ext}. These molecules will then have their H_A resonance at a slightly higher H_{ext} than would be expected in the absence of this coupling. In these molecules, the effect of the external magnetic field is diminished by the neighboring X proton; the $H_{coupling}$ of Equation 3-1 is negative.

The splitting of the X resonance by the coupling with the neighboring A proton is interpreted similarly. For that half of the molecules in which the A proton is oriented with H_{ext}, the resonance of the X proton will occur at a slightly lower value of H_{ext} than would be expected in the absence of coupling. For that half of the molecules in which the A proton is oriented against H_{ext}, the resonance of the X proton will occur at a slightly higher value of H_{ext} than if there were no coupling.

In this example, as in most cases where the neighboring protons are on adjacent carbon atoms connected by a single bond that is free to rotate, the magnitude of this effect, the splitting, is about 7 Hz. The usual notation is $J = 7$ Hz.

The strength of coupling between magnetically active nuclei is independent of the size of the external magnetic field. This is in contrast to shielding and chemical shift differences ($\Delta\delta$), which are proportional to the size of H_{ext}. An example may serve to illustrate this. Suppose the NMR spectrum of a substance obtained with a 60 MHz instrument indicates a chemical shift difference, $\Delta\delta$, of 1 ppm (which in this case would equal 60 Hz) and a coupling constant, J, of 7 Hz. One would then expect the spectrum of the same compound obtained with a 100 MHz instrument to indicate a chemical shift difference, $\Delta\delta$, of 1 ppm (which this time would equal 100 Hz) but still a coupling constant, J, of 7 Hz. Thus line spacings due to coupling can be distinguished from those due to chemical shift differences by obtaining the spectrum at two different external fields. Spacings due to coupling will be invariant, but spacings due to chemical shift differences will be proportional to the strength of the external field.

It is important to remember that in this analysis the multiplicity of a particular resonance (the splitting pattern) is interpreted in terms of the effect of **neighboring** magnetically active nuclei. These magnetically active neighbors are usually protons, but they could be any nucleus with a magnetic moment, for example, ^{19}F, ^{13}C, or ^{31}P.

In the next three chapters we will consider in more detail the interpretation and prediction of experimentally observable splitting patterns in terms of coupling between magnetically active nuclei.

PROBLEMS

3.1. Which of the following compounds would be expected to show only a single peak in its proton NMR spectrum?

a. $CH_3-\overset{\overset{\displaystyle O}{\|}}{C}-CH_3$ acetone

b. CH_3-O-CH_3 dimethyl ether

c. $CH_3-\overset{\overset{\displaystyle O}{\|}}{C}-O-CH_3$ methyl acetate

d. CH_3I methyl iodide

e. $Br-CH_2-Br$ dibromomethane

f. $Cl-CH_2-Br$ chlorobromomethane

g. $Br-CH_2CH_2-Br$ 1,2-dibromoethane

h. $Cl-CH_2CH_2-Br$ 1-chloro-2-bromoethane

3.2. Which member of each of the following pairs of structural isomers would be expected to show only a single peak in its proton NMR spectrum?

a. CH_3-CCl_3 or $CH_2Cl-CHCl_2$

b.   or

c. $\underset{CH_3}{\overset{CH_3}{>}}C=CH_2$ or $\begin{matrix} CH_2-CH_2 \\ | \qquad | \\ CH_2-CH_2 \end{matrix}$

d. $Cl-CH_2CH_2-Cl$ or $CH_3-\overset{\overset{\displaystyle Cl}{|}}{\underset{\underset{\displaystyle Cl}{|}}{C}}-H$

e. $H_2C=C=CH_2$ or $CH_3-C\equiv C-H$

3.3. Which structural isomer(s) of the molecular formula given will show only one singlet in its proton NMR spectrum?

a. C_5H_{12} b. C_5H_{10} c. C_5H_8

d. C_4H_8 e. C_4H_6 f. C_4H_4

g. C_4H_2 h. C_2H_6O i. C_2H_4O

j. C_2H_2O k. $C_3H_6Cl_2$ l. $C_3H_4Cl_4$

m. $C_3H_4Cl_2$ n. $C_3H_3Cl_3$ o. $C_4H_8O_2$

3.4. Which isomer(s) in each set will show only a singlet in its proton NMR spectrum?
   a.   the isomeric butyl chlorides
   b.   the isomeric dichlorobenzenes
   c.   the isomeric trichlorobenzenes.
   d.   the isomeric trichlorocyclopropanes
   e.   the isomeric tetrachlorocyclobutanes
3.5. Calculate the expected chemical shift for the peak due to the methylene group in each of the following compounds.
   a. $Br-CH_2-Cl$ bromochloromethane

   b. $CH_3-O-\overset{\overset{O}{\|}}{C}-CH_2-\overset{\overset{O}{\|}}{C}-O-CH_3$ dimethyl malonate

   c. $CH_3-\overset{\overset{O}{\|}}{C}-O-CH_2-O-\overset{\overset{O}{\|}}{C}-CH_3$ diacetylmethane
   d. $CH_3-O-CH_2-O-CH_3$ dimethoxymethane

   e.   piperonal

3.6. How many Hertz does 1 ppm correspond to for an NMR spectrometer operating at a radiofrequency of
   a.   30 MHz?
   b.   100 MHz?
3.7. How many gauss does 1 ppm correspond to for a proton NMR spectrometer operating at a radiofrequency of
   a.   30 MHz?
   b.   100 MHz?
3.8. Since the difference in energy between two nuclear spin states, ΔE, is proportional to the magnetic field experienced by the nuclei, what gain in sensitivity can be achieved by using a 300 MHz spectrometer rather than a 60 MHz spectrometer? (See Equations 2-1 and 2-2; sensitivity is proportional to the fractional excess of nuclei in the ground state.)
3.9. According to Table 2-1, how many ppm distant from a typical proton resonance is a typical ^{19}F resonance?
3.10. The proton NMR spectrum of each of the following compounds consists of two peaks (two singlets). Predict the relative intensities of the two peaks.
   a. $CH_3-\overset{\overset{O}{\|}}{C}-O-CH_3$ methyl acetate

b. $CH_3-O-CH_2-C\equiv N$ methoxyacetonitrile

c. $CH_3-O-\overset{\overset{O}{\|}}{C}-CH_2-\overset{\overset{O}{\|}}{C}-O-CH_3$ dimethyl malonate

d. $CH_3-O-CH_2CH_2-O-CH_3$ 1,2-dimethoxyethane

e.

p-dimethoxybenzene

4 First-Order Splitting Patterns: The $N+1$ Rule

In Chapter 3 we briefly described three characteristics of NMR spectra which can yield information about the sample: the chemical shift, the integral, and the splitting pattern. In this chapter we will further develop the model for the interpretation of splitting patterns that was introduced in the preceding section.

4.1 ONE ISOLATED SET OF NUCLEI: A_n SYSTEMS

If all the magnetically active nuclei in a molecule have exactly the same chemical shift, their resonance will appear as a single peak, a *singlet*. We have already seen two examples of this: benzene (Figure 3-1) and 1,1,2,2-tetrachloroethane (Figure 3-5). Although the splitting of the resonances of 1,1-dibromo-2,2-dichloroethane (Figure 3-6) was interpreted in terms of coupling between the two protons, it appears from the spectrum of 1,1,2,2-tetrachloroethane that such coupling is not manifest as splitting when the nuclei all have the same chemical shift. The situation is similar with benzene. Although later we will interpret the spectra of some benzene derivatives in terms of coupling among the ring protons, it appears that in the case of benzene itself such coupling does not result in splitting. The reason is that all six ring protons have the same chemical shift.

According to this reasoning, we would expect the spectra of methyl iodide, 1,1,1-trichloroethane, and 1,2-dichloroethane each to consist of one singlet, since in each molecule all the protons should have exactly the same chemical shift. The spectra of these molecules, shown in Figures 4-1 through 4-3, confirm this expectation.

$$
\begin{array}{c}
\text{H} \\
| \\
\text{H}-\text{C}-\text{I} \\
| \\
\text{H}
\end{array}
$$

methyl iodide

$$
\begin{array}{cc}
\text{Cl} & \text{H} \\
| & | \\
\text{Cl}-\text{C}-\text{C}-\text{H} \\
| & | \\
\text{Cl} & \text{H}
\end{array}
$$

1,1,1-trichloroethane

$$
\begin{array}{cc}
\text{H} & \text{H} \\
| & | \\
\text{Cl}-\text{C}-\text{C}-\text{Cl} \\
| & | \\
\text{H} & \text{H}
\end{array}
$$

1,2-dichloroethane

Even if all the protons in a molecule do not have the same chemical shift, it is sometimes possible for them to occur in sets that are sufficiently isolated from one another that they can be considered independently. For example, the proton NMR spectrum of methyl acetate shows two singlets (Figure 4-4).

$$
\begin{array}{c}
\overset{1.55}{} \quad \overset{\text{O}}{\underset{||}{}} \quad \overset{2.50}{} \\
\text{CH}_3-\text{C}-\text{O}-\text{CH}_3
\end{array}
$$

methyl acetate

Apparently the coupling *between* the protons of each set—*interset coupling*—is essentially zero, and therefore the two sets of three protons can be considered separately. Each three-proton set gives a singlet, because within each set all protons have the same chemical shift. Any coupling among the protons *within* each set—*intraset coupling*—will not be manifest as splitting.

Figure 4-1   Proton NMR Spectrum of Methyl Iodide; CCl₄ Solution.

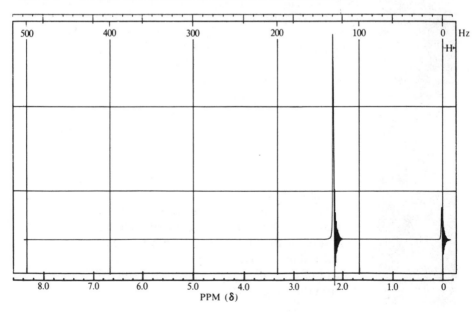

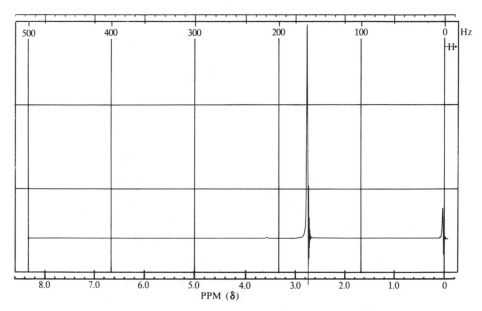

Figure 4-2   Proton NMR Spectrum of 1,1,1-Trichloroethane; CCl₄ Solution.

Figure 4-3   Proton NMR Spectrum of 1,2-Dichloroethane; CCl₄ Solution.

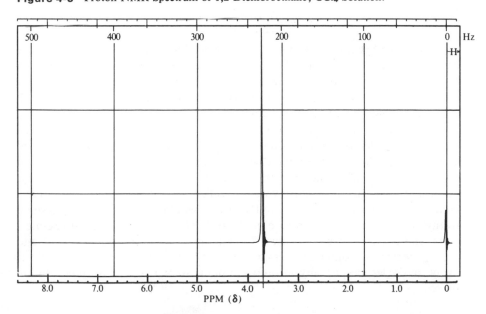

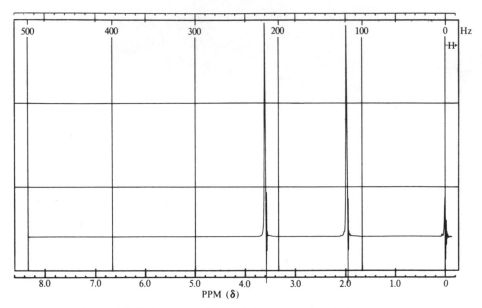

Figure 4-4 Proton NMR Spectrum of Methyl Acetate; CCl₄ Solution.

The spectrum of para-xylene (Figure 3-2) may be interpreted in a similar

$$CH_3$$

H   H

H   H

$$CH_3$$

para-xylene

way. Each methyl group makes up an independent three-proton set, and the four ring protons form a third independent set. Because of the symmetry of the molecule, the two methyl singlets will have exactly the same chemical shift and will appear as a single peak of relative area six, and the ring protons will appear as a singlet of relative area four.

In terms of a notation that is often used to describe sets of coupled magnetically active nuclei, the examples discussed in this section could all be described as A_n systems, where n is the number of magnetically active nuclei with chemical shift A. Thus 1,1,2,2-tetrachloroethane would be called an A_2 system, methyl iodide and 1,1,1-trichloroethane would be called A_3 systems, 1,2-dichloroethane would be called an A_4 system, and benzene would be called an A_6 system. Methyl acetate would be said to contain two A_3 systems at different chemical shifts, and p-xylene to contain two A_3 systems at the same chemical shift and one A_4 system at a different chemical shift. The resonance of an A_n system is always a singlet. despite any intraset coupling among the n members within the set.

Other molecules that provide examples of one or more A_n spin systems and whose proton NMR spectra consist of one singlet include p-dichlorobenzene (A_4), ethane (A_6), cyclohexane (A_{12}), acetone (two A_3 systems), dioxane (two A_4 systems), tert-butyl bromide (three A_3 systems), and tetramethylsilane (four A_3 systems).

p-dichlorobenzene   ethane   cyclohexane

acetone   dioxane   tert-butyl   TMS
                                bromide

In order for sets of protons to be independent of one another they must be separated by four or more single bonds. Thus protons on either the same or adjacent atoms would be expected to be coupled, but protons on atoms separated by a third atom would not be expected to be coupled:

$$H-C-H \qquad \text{coupling} > 0$$
$$H-C-C-H \qquad \text{coupling} > 0$$
$$H-C-C-C-H \qquad \text{coupling} \cong 0$$

Multiple bonds appear to be better " conductors " of coupling than single bonds. The relationships between the magnitude of coupling and molecular structure will be considered in more detail in Chapter 7.

4.2   TWO COUPLED SETS OF NUCLEI: A_nX_m SYSTEMS

If two sets of magnetically active nuclei, each at a different chemical shift, are not sufficiently isolated from one another, their resonances will appear as multiple peaks—a *multiplet*—rather than as singlets. The spacings between the peaks of the multiplet will be determined by the strength of the coupling between the nuclei of the two sets, the *interset coupling*. The case of 1,1-dibromo-2,2-dichloroethane, described in Section 3.1, is an example of this. Apparently the

1,1-dibromo-2,2-dichloroethane

A proton and the *X* proton are not sufficiently isolated from one another to be considered separately since the resonance of each (Figure 3-6) appears as a doublet. The spacing between the members of each doublet, 7 Hz, equals the magnitude of the coupling between the two protons. In this case the interset coupling constant, J_{AX}, equals 7 Hz. In Section 3.3, the appearance of each resonance as a 1 : 1 doublet was interpreted in terms of the proton of one set either augmenting or diminishing the strength of the external magnetic field for the proton of the other set.

The molecule 1,1,2-trichloroethane is another case where protons at

$$\begin{array}{cc} \text{Cl} & \text{H}_X \\ | & | \\ \text{H}_A{-}\text{C}{-}\text{C}{-}\text{Cl} \\ | & | \\ \text{Cl} & \text{H}_X \end{array}$$

1,1,2-trichloroethane

different chemical shifts, the *A* proton and the *X* protons, cannot be considered separately. As shown in Figure 4-5, the resonance of the *A* proton appears as a 1 : 2 : 1 triplet and the resonance of the *X* protons as a 1 : 1 doublet. The total area of the resonance of the doublet is twice that of the triplet. The resonance of the *A* proton is split into a 1 : 2 : 1 triplet through coupling with the two neighboring *X* protons at a different chemical shift, and the resonance of the *X* protons is split into a 1 : 1 doublet through coupling with the one neighboring *A* proton. The spacing of the members of each multiplet is approximately 7 Hz which means that the interset coupling constant, J_{AX}, is about 7 Hz.

Figure 4-5 Proton NMR Spectrum of 1,1,2-Trichloroethane; CCl$_4$ Solution.

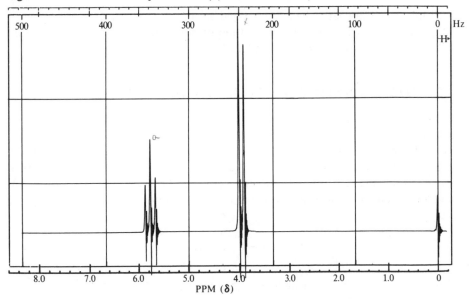

The splitting patterns of this example can also be interpreted in terms of the model presented in Section 3.3. The resonance of the X protons appears as two equal peaks (a 1 : 1 doublet) because in half the molecules, H_A will be oriented with the external magnetic field (↑) and will augment it, and in the other half of the molecules, H_A will be oriented against the external field (↓) and will diminish it. The X protons of half the molecules will absorb rf energy at a lower value of H_{ext}, and the remainder will absorb energy at a higher value of H_{ext}.

The resonance of the A proton appears as an evenly spaced triplet whose members have a relative intensity of 1 : 2 : 1; the reason is that for one-fourth of the molecules the neighboring X protons will both be oriented with the external field (↑↑), for one-half the molecules one neighboring X proton will be oriented with and one against the external field (↑↓ and ↓↑), and for one-fourth of the molecules the neighboring X protons will both be oriented against the external field (↓↓). Therefore the A protons of one-fourth of the molecules will absorb rf energy at a value of H_{ext} slightly lower than if the X protons were not there, the A protons of one-half of the molecules will absorb rf energy at the same value of H_{ext} as they would if the X protons were not there, since for these molecules the X protons eliminate one another's effect, and the A protons of one-fourth of the molecules will absorb rf energy at a slightly higher value of H_{ext} than if the X protons were not there.

Notice that the possible intraset coupling constant, J_{XX}, has not been mentioned in this interpretation; the splitting pattern is determined *only* by the interset coupling constant, J_{AX}.

The protons of 1,1,2-trichloroethane can be described as an AX_2 spin system. This notation means that there is one magnetically active nucleus at chemical shift A and two at a very different chemical shift X. In addition, it is also implied that each of the two possible interset coupling constants, J_{AX}, are exactly the same. This latter condition we will call *magnetic equivalence*.

Another example of an AX_2 (or $A_2 X$) spin system is the molecule 1,1,2,3,3-pentachloropropane. For this molecule the proton NMR spectrum (Figure 4-6)

$$\begin{array}{ccccc} & Cl & H_A & Cl & \\ & | & | & | & \\ H_X-C & -C & -C & -H_X \\ & | & | & | & \\ & Cl & Cl & Cl & \end{array}$$

1,1,2,3,3-pentachloropropane

shows a 1 : 1 doublet for the two X protons, and a 1 : 2 : 1 triplet for the A proton. The total area of the doublet is twice that of the triplet. The interpretation of the spectrum of this compound is exactly analogous to that for the spectrum of 1,1,2-trichloroethane.

The proton NMR spectrum of 1,2-dichloroethane was shown in Figure 3-4 to be a singlet. The NMR spectrum of the structurally isomeric 1,1-dichloroethane shows a 1 : 1 doublet and a 1 : 3 : 3 : 1 quartet (Figure 4-7). The resonance of the methyl protons (the X protons) appears as a 1 : 1 doublet of relative

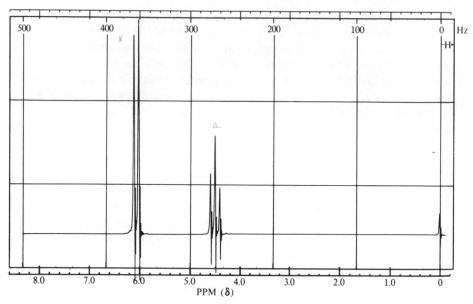

Figure 4-6   Proton NMR Spectrum of 1,1,2,3,3-Pentachloropropane; CCl_4 Solution.

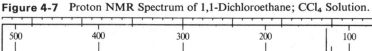

Figure 4-7   Proton NMR Spectrum of 1,1-Dichloroethane; CCl_4 Solution.

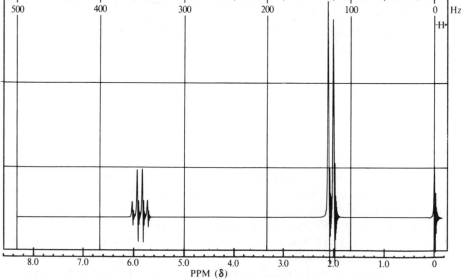

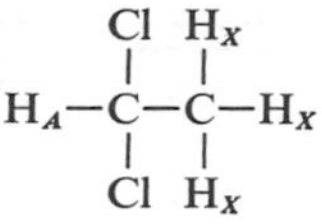

$$\underset{\text{1,1-dichloroethane}}{\begin{array}{c} \text{Cl } \text{H}_X \\ | \quad | \\ \text{H}_A{-}\text{C}{-}\text{C}{-}\text{H}_X \\ | \quad | \\ \text{Cl } \text{H}_X \end{array}}$$

intensity 3 due to coupling with the A proton. The resonance of the A proton appears as a $1:3:3:1$ quartet of relative intensity 1 due to coupling with the three X protons. The resonance of the A proton appears as a $1:3:3:1$ quartet because the three neighboring X protons can be oriented either all three with the external field ($\uparrow\uparrow\uparrow$; one-eighth of the molecules), or two with and one against ($\uparrow\uparrow\downarrow$, $\uparrow\downarrow\uparrow$, $\downarrow\uparrow\uparrow$; three-eighths of the molecules) or one with and two against ($\uparrow\downarrow\downarrow$, $\downarrow\uparrow\downarrow$, $\downarrow\downarrow\uparrow$; three-eighths of the molecules) or all three against ($\downarrow\downarrow\downarrow$; one-eighth of the molecules). The resonance of the three X protons again appears as a $1:1$ doublet because the neighboring A proton can be oriented either with or against the external magnetic field. This molecule can be classified as an example of an AX_3 (or A_3X) spin system.

All the examples described in this section can be classified as A_nX_m spin systems. This notation means that there are n magnetically active nuclei with chemical shift A and m magnetically active nuclei with quite a different chemical shift X, and all (n times m) possible J_{AX} values are exactly the same (magnetic equivalence is involved). The magnetically active A and X nuclei are otherwise isolated from any other magnetically active nuclei in the molecule. When this is the case, the splitting patterns for the A and X nuclei will follow the "$N+1$ Rule."* This rule has two parts. First, the **number of peaks** in the multiplet for the resonance of one set of nuclei will be one more than the number of nuclei in the other set. Second, the **relative intensities** of the peaks within the multiplet will follow the coefficients of the binomial distribution: doublets will be $1:1$, triplets will be $1:2:1$, quartets will be $1:3:3:1$, quintets will be $1:4:6:4:1$, and so on as indicated in Figure 4-8. This has been the case with all the examples described in this section.

Figure 4-8   The $N+1$ Rule

Number of neighbors	Number of peaks in multiplet	Name of multiplet	Relative intensities within multiplet
0	1	singlet	1
1	2	doublet	$1:1$
2	3	triplet	$1:2:1$
3	4	quartet	$1:3:3:1$
4	5	quintet	$1:4:6:4:1$
5	6	sextet	$1:5:10:10:5:1$
6	7	septet	$1:6:15:20:15:6:1$
$\vdots$	$\vdots$	$\vdots$	$\vdots$
N	$N+1$		

---

* This is a specific case of a more general rule involving nuclei other than protons.

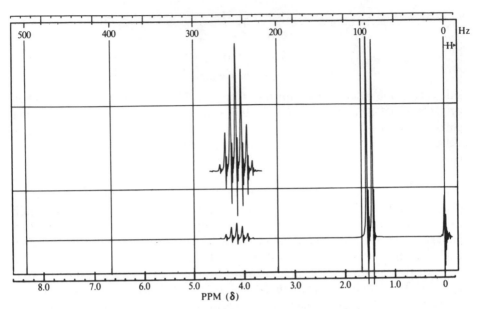

500   400   300   200   100   0 Hz

8.0   7.0   6.0   5.0   4.0   3.0   2.0   1.0   0

PPM (δ)

Figure 4-9   Proton NMR Spectrum of 2-Chloropropane; CCl₄ Solution.

We end this section with two more examples of molecules that contain $A_n X_m$ systems. The first is 2-chloropropane. According to the $N + 1$ Rule we

H—C—C—C—H

2-chloropropane

would expect the six methyl protons to appear as a 1 : 1 doublet due to coupling with the single proton on the carbon bearing the chlorine atom. We would also expect the single proton to appear as a 1 : 6 : 15 : 20 : 15 : 6 : 1 septet due to coupling with the six methyl protons. The spectrum of 2-chloropropane is shown in Figure 4-9 and its appearance is consistent with these expectations. The inset shows the septet rescanned at a higher spectrum amplitude so that the weak outer peaks can be seen. Since there are six methyl protons, the total intensity of the doublet is six times that of the septet.

The final example is 1-chloroethane. According to the $N + 1$ Rule we would

H—C—C—Cl

1-chloroethane

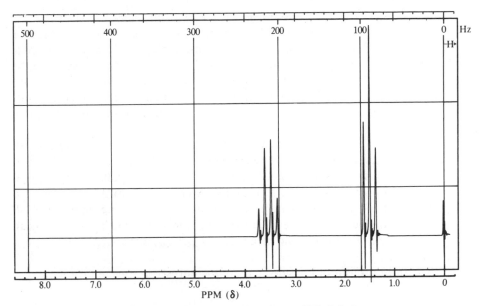

Figure 4-10   Proton NMR Spectrum of 1-Chloroethane; CCl_4 Solution.

expect the methyl resonance to appear as a $1 : 2 : 1$ triplet due to coupling with the two neighboring methylene protons, and the methylene resonance to appear as a $1 : 3 : 3 : 1$ quartet due to coupling with the three neighboring methyl protons. The spectrum (Figure 4-10) is in agreement with these expectations and is a good example of the typical "ethyl resonance." The relative intensities of the triplet and quartet are as three is to two.

It should be apparent that the spectra of A_n systems are also consistent with the $N + 1$ Rule. With no magnetically active neighbors their resonances should be a one line "multiplet."

4.3   EXTENSIONS OF THE $N + 1$ RULE

As we have now seen, the $N + 1$ Rule describes the appearance of the NMR spectra of molecules whose magnetically active nuclei give resonances at two different chemical shifts, providing that two conditions are met. First, all possible interset coupling constants must be equal (all J_{AX} must have the same value; magnetic equivalence is involved). Second, the difference in chemical shift between the two sets of nuclei, $\Delta\delta$, must be large relative to the interset coupling constant, J_{AX} (i.e., $\Delta\delta/J_{AX}$ must be of the order of 10 or greater).

In this section we shall describe how the $N + 1$ Rule can be extended to systems involving magnetically active nuclei at three or more different chemical shifts. Then, in Chapters 5 and 6, we shall describe NMR spectra of molecules for which one or the other of the two conditions just stated is not met.

If the molecular structure and geometry of a substance are such that its magnetically active nuclei would be expected to give resonances at three or more different chemical shifts, the two conditions that must be met in order for the spectrum to be interpretable in terms of an extended $N + 1$ Rule are the following: (1) all interset coupling constants of each type must be equal (magnetic equivalence must be involved), and (2) the difference in chemical shift between sets of nuclei must be large relative to the corresponding coupling constant.

If these conditions were met by a molecule in which the magnetically active nuclei gave resonances at three different chemical shifts, it would be classified as an $A_n M_p X_m$ system. This would mean that there were n nuclei with chemical shift, A, p with chemical shift M, and m with chemical shift X. It would also mean that all possible J_{AM} were equal, all possible J_{MX} were equal, and all possible J_{AX} were equal; magnetic equivalence is involved. (This does not mean $J_{AM} = J_{AX}$, etc.). Finally it would mean that $\Delta\delta_{AM}/J_{AM}$, $\Delta\delta_{MX}/J_{MX}$, and $\Delta\delta_{AX}/J_{AX}$ were all large.

The three protons of the side-chain of p-chlorostyrene make up a system of

p-chlorostyrene

this type, an $A_1 M_1 X_1$ system, or simply an AMX system. The proton NMR spectrum of this compound is shown in Figure 4-11, and the inset shows an enlargement of the part of the spectrum due to the side-chain. The twelve line spectrum is best described as three pairs of doublets; one pair of doublets corresponds to each of the three protons. The extended $N + 1$ Rule interpretation of this splitting pattern is that the resonance of the A proton is split into a doublet by coupling with the M proton and then further split into a pair of doublets by coupling with the X proton. Similarly, the resonance of the M proton is split into a doublet by coupling with the A proton and then further split into a pair of doublets by coupling with the X proton. The appearance of the resonance of the X proton is similarly accounted for in terms of successive splitting by the A and M protons. In this interpretation of the splitting pattern of the A proton, for example, it makes no difference whether you consider first the effect of the M proton and then the X proton, or vice versa. Figure 4-12 shows that the two approaches are exactly equivalent.

In Chapter 7 we will consider this spectrum again and see how the values for the three interset coupling constants can be obtained from the spacings of the multiplets.

It should be apparent that the condition of magnetic equivalence was automatically met in this case since there was only one magnetically active nucleus at each different chemical shift.

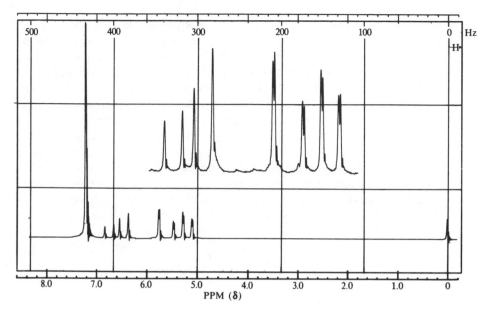

Figure 4-11   Proton NMR Spectrum of *p*-Chlorostyrene; CCl₄ Solution.

Figure 4-12   Prediction of the Appearance of the Resonance of a Nucleus, A, Split by $J_{AM} = 6$ Hz and $J_{AX} = 4$ Hz.

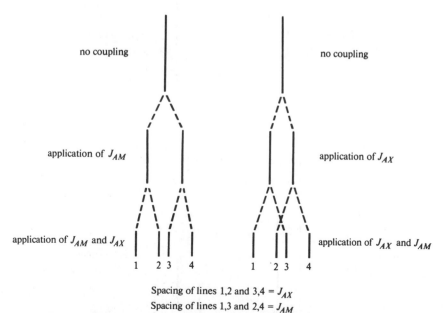

no coupling   no coupling

application of J_{AM} application of J_{AX}

application of J_{AM} and J_{AX} application of J_{AX} and J_{AM}

1   2 3   4   1   2 3   4

Spacing of lines 1,2 and 3,4 = J_{AX}
Spacing of lines 1,3 and 2,4 = J_{AM}

In the above example, the resonance of the A proton appeared as a pair of doublets. Earlier we saw that the A proton of an AX_2 system would appear as a $1:2:1$ triplet. The AX_2 system may also be considered to be a special case of the AMX system in which A and M have the same chemical shift and $J_{AX} = J_{MX}$, as shown in Figure 4-13. From this point of view, a $1:2:1$ triplet is seen to be a special case of a pair of doublets in which the couplings to the other two magnetically active nuclei are exactly the same so that the inner lines of each pair of doublets coincide to give a single line twice as intense as the other two. Actually, all regular $N + 1$ Rule multiplets may also be considered to be built up by the process of successive splitting by equally coupled neighbors.

An example of an AMX system in which all three interset coupling constants are essentially equal and each multiplet appears as a $1:2:1$ triplet is that of 1-bromo-3-chloro-5-iodobenzene (Figure 4-14).

1-bromo-3-chloro-5-iodobenzene

Figure 4-13   Prediction of the Appearance of the Resonance of an $A_2 X$ System as a Special Case of an AMX System for which $\Delta\delta_{AM} = 0$ and $J_{AX} = J$.

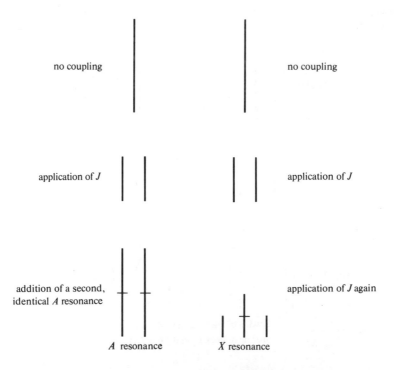

no coupling   no coupling

application of J application of J

addition of a second, identical A resonance   application of J again

A resonance X resonance

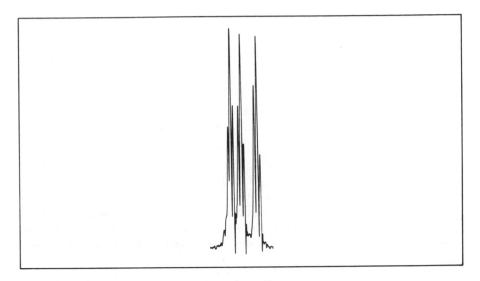

Figure 4-14 Proton NMR Spectrum of 1-Bromo-3-chloro-5-iodobenzene; CCl₄ Solution.

In an *AMX* system, it is possible for one of the coupling constants to be very small or zero. When this happens, the resonance of only one magnetically active nucleus appears as a *pair* of doublets; the resonances of the other two appear only as doublets (8 lines in all). The spectrum of such a system, that of 2,4-dinitrochlorobenzene, is shown in Figure 4-15. The resonance of the *A*

Figure 4-15 Proton NMR Spectrum of 2,4-Dinitrochlorobenzene; CCl₄ Solution. Offset = 1 δ

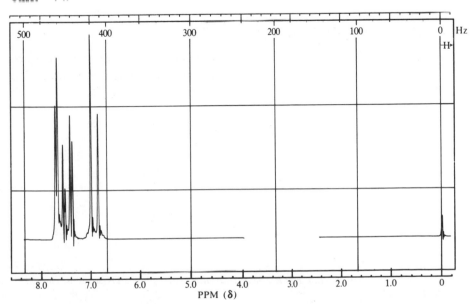

2,4-dinitrochlorobenzene

proton appears as the left-hand doublet, the resonance of the X proton appears as the right-hand doublet, and the resonance of the M proton appears as the middle pair of doublets. In this case $J_{para} = 0$, and the assignment of resonances was made assuming that J_{ortho} was greater than J_{meta} as is generally the case.

If there is more than one magnetically active nucleus at each chemical shift, the appearance of the NMR spectrum can be predicted by this extension of the $N + 1$ Rule. For example, the proton NMR spectrum of 2-butenoic acid-γ-lactone would be predicted to appear as follows: the resonance of the A

2-butenoic acid-γ-lactone

proton should appear as a pair of 1 : 2 : 1 triplets (by successive splitting by the two X protons and the one M proton), that of the M proton also as a pair of triplets, and that of the two X protons as a pair of doublets. The appearance of the spectrum agrees very well with this prediction.*

4.4 SUMMARY OF THE $N + 1$ RULE

In this chapter we have considered examples in which it is possible to interpret the spin-spin splitting pattern of the NMR spectrum in a simple way, according to the $N + 1$ Rule. The various possibilities that have been discussed can be summarized as follows.

	Appearance of Resonance
A. Spin System	A Resonance
A	singlet
A_2	singlet
A_3	singlet
$\vdots$	$\vdots$
A_m	singlet

---

* Spectrum 51, *High Resolution NMR Spectra Catalog*, vol. 1, Varian Associates, Palo Alto, California, 1962.

Appearance of Resonance

B. Spin System	A Resonance	X Resonance
AX	$1:1$ doublet	$1:1$ doublet
AX_2	$1:2:1$ triplet	$1:1$ doublet
AX_3	$1:3:3:1$ quartet	$1:1$ doublet
⋮	⋮	⋮
AX_n	$(n+1)$-memb. multiplet	$1:1$ doublet
$A_2 X_2$	$1:2:1$ triplet	$1:2:1$ triplet
$A_2 X_3$	$1:3:3:1$ quartet	$1:2:1$ triplet
⋮	⋮	⋮
$A_2 X_n$	$(n+1)$-memb. multiplet	$1:2:1$ triplet
⋮	⋮	⋮
$A_m X_n$	$(n+1)$-memb. multiplet	$(m+1)$-memb. multiplet

Appearance of Resonance

C. Spin System	A Resonance	M Resonance	X Resonance
AMX	pair of doublets	pair of doublets	pair of doublets
AMX_2	pair of triplets	pair of triplets	pair of doublets
AMX_3	pair of quartets	pair of quartets	pair of doublets
⋮	⋮	⋮	⋮
$A_m M_p X_n$	$(p+1)$ of $(n+1)$	$(m+1)$ of $(n+1)$	$(m+1)$ of $(p+1)$

PROBLEMS

4.1. Identify each of the A_n spin systems in the following compounds. Indicate which A_n spin systems will have exactly the same chemical shift. Predict the number and relative intensities of the singlets expected for each proton NMR spectrum.

a.
$$
\begin{array}{cc}
\text{O} & \text{CH}_3 \\
\parallel & \mid \\
\text{CH}_3-\text{C}-\text{C}-\text{CH}_3 \\
& \mid \\
& \text{CH}_3
\end{array}
$$

b.
$$
\begin{array}{c}
\text{CH}_3 \\
\mid \\
\text{CH}_3-\text{O}-\text{CH}_2-\text{C}-\text{CH}_3 \\
\mid \\
\text{CH}_3
\end{array}
$$

c. $\text{CH}_3-\text{O}-\text{CH}_2-$⟨benzene ring⟩$-\text{CH}_2-\text{O}-\text{CH}_3$

d.
$$
\begin{array}{c}
\text{CH}_2-\text{Br} \\
\mid \\
\text{CH}_3-\text{C}-\text{CH}_2-\text{Br} \\
\mid \\
\text{CH}_3
\end{array}
$$

e.

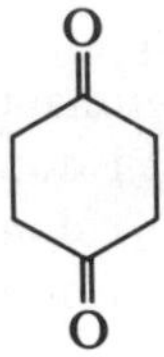

f.

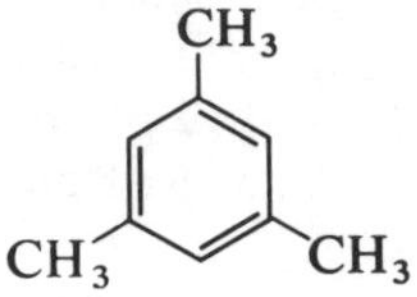

g.

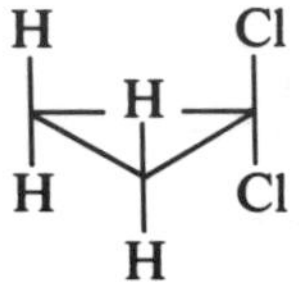

4.2. Assume that the $N + 1$ Rule applies. Predict the appearance of the proton NMR spectrum of each of the following compounds. How many multiplets will be observed? What will be their relative intensities? What will be the relative intensities of the individual peaks within each multiplet?

a. $Br-CH_2CHCl_2$

b. CH_3-CH_2-Br

c. $Cl_2CH-CH_2-CHCl_2$

d.

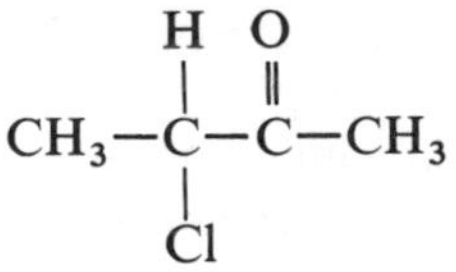

e.

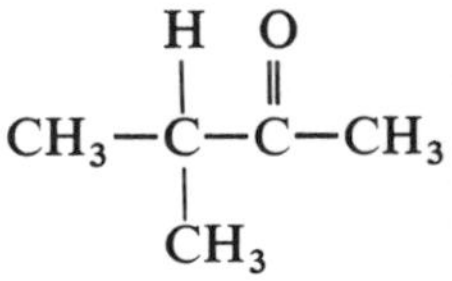

f. 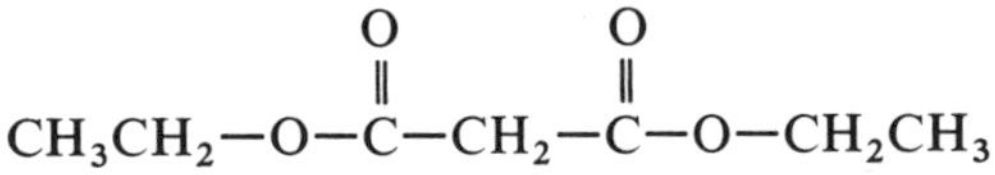 $CH_3CH_2-O-\overset{\overset{O}{\|}}{C}-CH_2-\overset{\overset{O}{\|}}{C}-O-CH_2CH_3$

g.

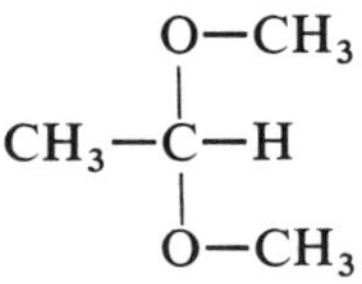

h. 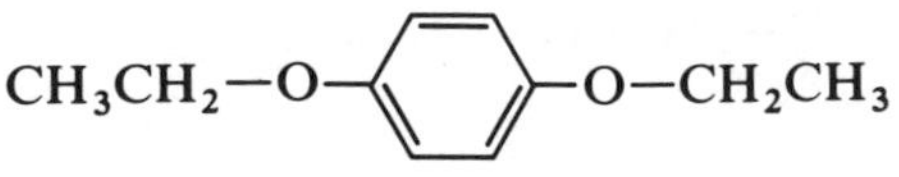 CH_3CH_2-O- $-O-CH_2CH_3$

i. 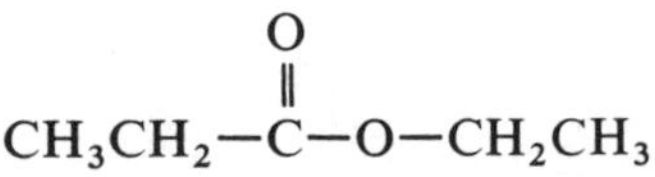 $CH_3CH_2-\overset{\overset{O}{\|}}{C}-O-CH_2CH_3$

4.3. Assume that the extended $N + 1$ Rule applies. Predict the appearance of the proton NMR spectrum of each of the following compounds. How many multiplets will be observed? What will be their relative intensities? What will be the relative intensities of the individual peaks within each multiplet?

a.

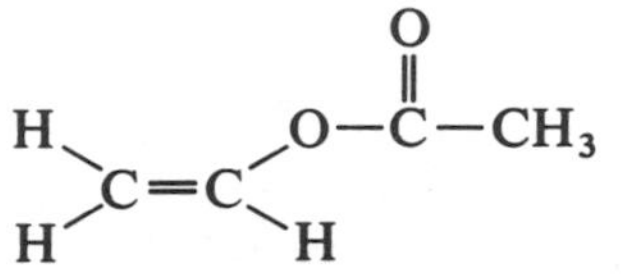

The methyl protons make up an independent A_3 system. Varian 65*; compare with Figure 7-6.

b.

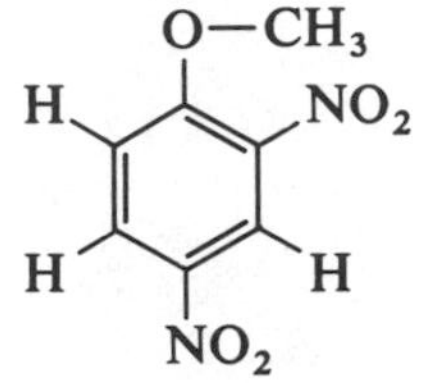

The methyl protons make up an independent A_3 system. Varian 149*

c.

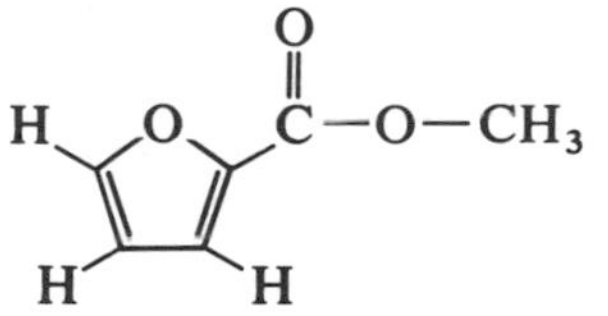

The methyl protons make up an independent A_3 system. Varian 125*

d.

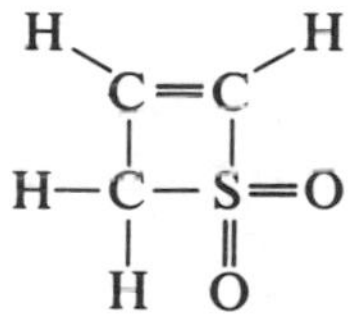

Varian 22*

e.

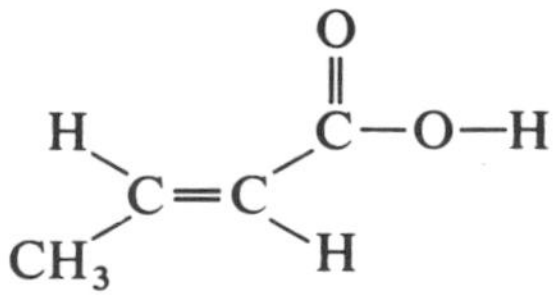

The carboxyl proton makes up an independent A_1 system. Varian 61*

f.

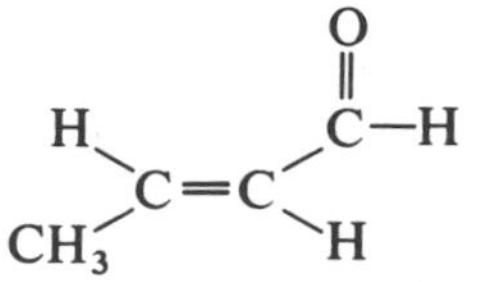

Varian 60*

---

* The reference is to the spectrum number in the *High Resolution NMR Spectra Catalog*, vol. 1, Varian Associates, Palo Alto, California, 1962.

5 Distorted First-Order Splitting Patterns: $\Delta\delta$ Not Large Relative to J

In Chapter 4 a number of examples of NMR spectra were presented in which it was possible to interpret the splitting patterns in a simple way, according to the $N + 1$ Rule. It was mentioned at that time, however, that two conditions must be met in order for the $N + 1$ Rule to apply. First, all coupling constants between members of two sets of magnetically active nuclei at different chemical shifts must be equal; magnetic equivalence is involved. Second, the one interset coupling constant, J, must be small relative to the corresponding chemical shift difference, $\Delta\delta$, between the two sets of magnetically active nuclei. In this chapter, we will see what the consequences are if the second condition is not met. (The consequences of failure to meet the first condition will be discussed in Chapter 6.)

5.1 TWO COUPLED SETS OF NUCLEI

An example of an NMR spectrum in which the splitting patterns cannot be accounted for by the $N + 1$ Rule is that of 1,2,3-trichlorobenzene. According to the $N + 1$ rule, the resonance of the middle proton should appear as a $1 : 2 : 1$ triplet, and that of the other two protons as a $1 : 1$ doublet (five lines in all). The spectrum actually shows a total of seven lines (Figure 5-1). The reason is that the chemical shift difference between the two resonances, $\Delta\delta$, is too small relative to the interset coupling constant, J—the $\Delta\delta/J$ ratio is too small.

$$\text{1,2,3-trichlorobenzene}$$

Although the $N + 1$ Rule cannot account for the splitting pattern in this case, the methods of quantum mechanics are able to do so. Figure 5-2 shows some of the results of such quantum mechanical calculations. From the figure you can see that if $\Delta\delta$ is sufficiently large relative to J (i.e., if the $\Delta\delta/J$ ratio is large), the results of the $N + 1$ Rule and of quantum mechanical calculations are about the same. However, as $\Delta\delta$ decreases relative to J, only the results of quantum mechanical calculations resemble the observed spectrum.

The situation is similar for the other $A_m X_n$ systems; Figure 5-3 shows examples of the calculated spacings and relative intensities for the AX system as a function of the decreasing $\Delta\delta/J$ ratio. As $\Delta\delta/J$ decreases because $\Delta\delta$ becomes smaller, the resonances move closer together, the inner lines grow, and the outer lines shrink. Figures 5-4, 5-5, and 5-6 show some of the results of quantum mechanical calculations for the AX_3, $A_2 X_2$, and $A_2 X_3$ systems. As $\Delta\delta/J$ decreases, the resonances move together, more lines appear, the inner lines become more intense, and the outer ones fade away. At the limit where $\Delta\delta$ goes to zero, the inner lines all coincide and the outer ones all disappear to give a

Figure 5-1   Proton NMR Spectrum of 1,2,3-Trichlorobenzene; CCl_4 Solution.

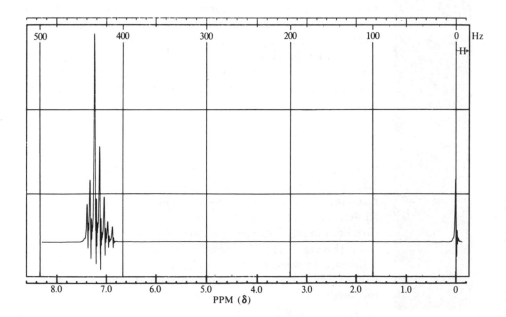

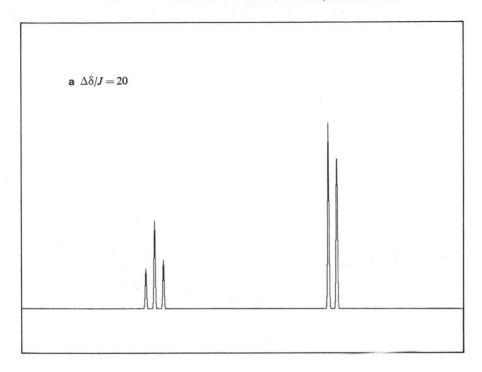

a $\Delta\delta/J = 20$

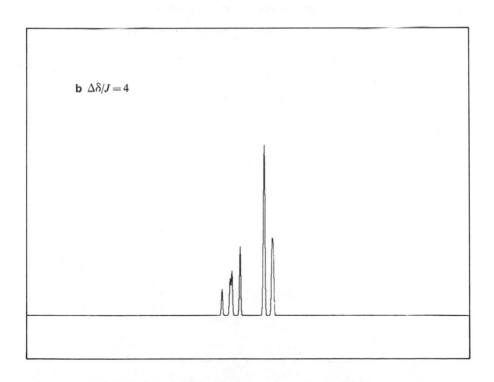

b $\Delta\delta/J = 4$

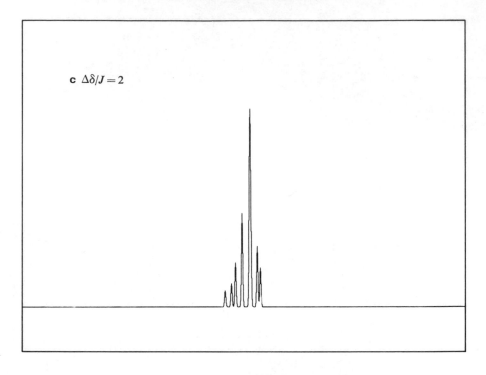

c $\Delta\delta/J = 2$

Figures 5-2a, b, and c   Calculated Spectra for the $AX_2\text{-}AB_2$ System.

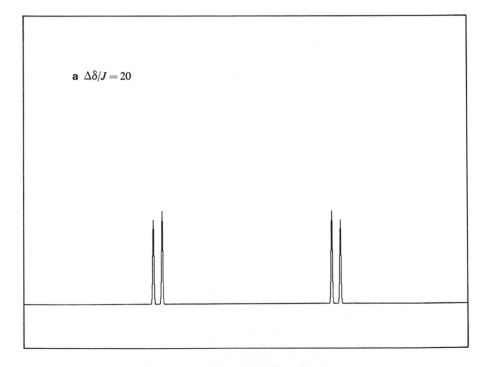

a $\Delta\delta/J = 20$

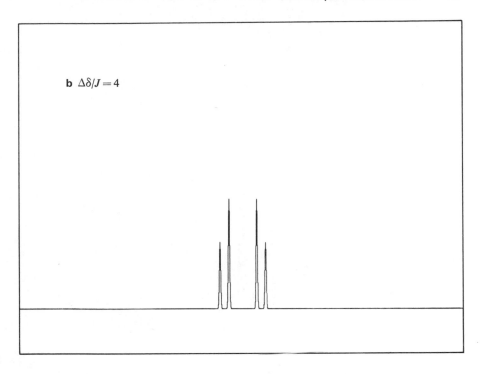

b $\Delta\delta/J = 4$

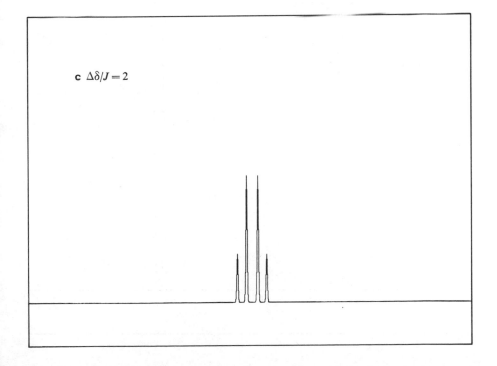

c $\Delta\delta/J = 2$

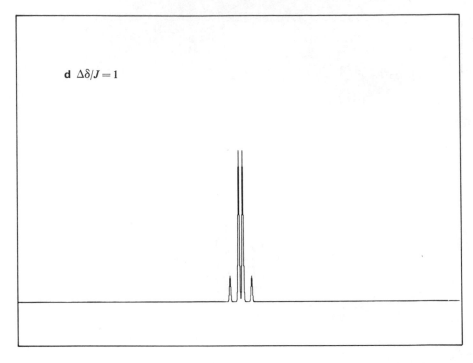

d $\Delta\delta/J = 1$

Figures 5-3a, b, c, and d   Calculated Spectra for the AX-AB System.

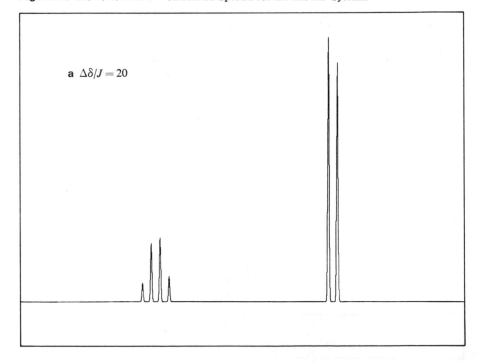

a $\Delta\delta/J = 20$

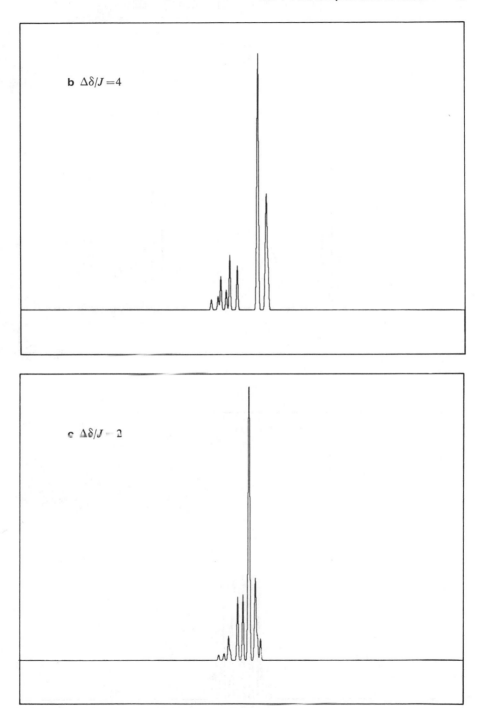

Figures 5-4a, b, and c   Calculated Spectra for the AX_3-AB_3 System.

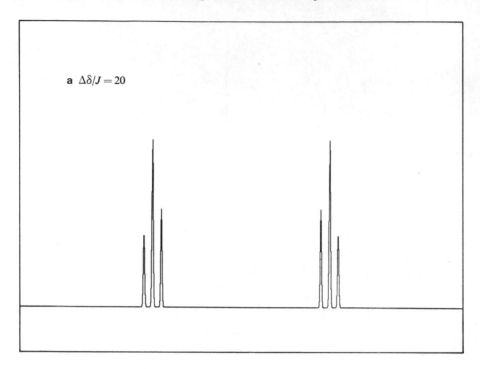

a $\Delta\delta/J = 20$

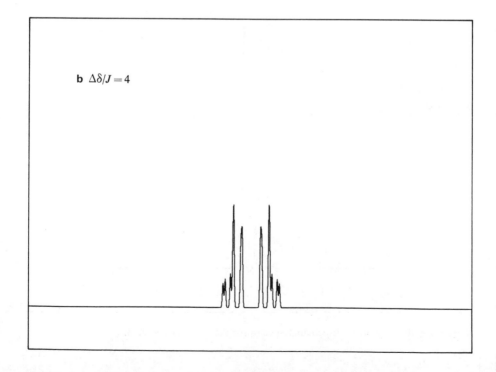

b $\Delta\delta/J = 4$

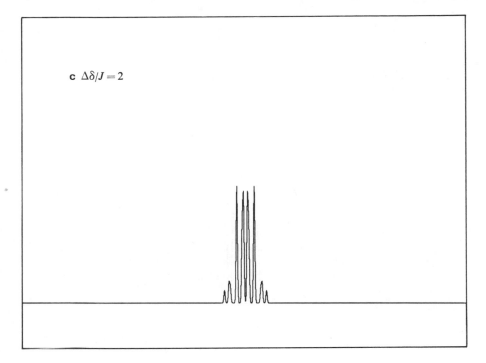

Figures 5-5 a, b, and c   Calculated Spectra for the $A_2 X_2$-$A_2 B_2$ System.

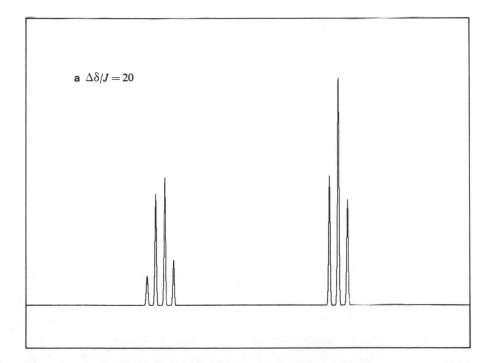

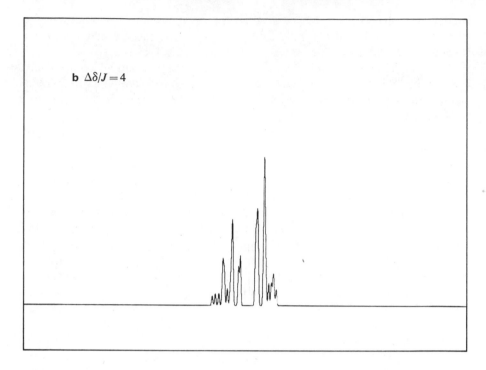

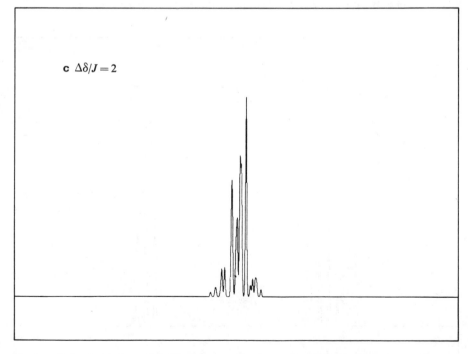

Figures 5-6a, b, and c   Calculated Spectra for the $A_2 X_3$-$A_2 B_3$ System.

singlet (just what the $N + 1$ Rule predicts for an A_n system). The intermediate cases are often referred to as AB, AB_2, etc. systems; the use of letters close together in the alphabet implies small chemical shift differences.

Although the $N + 1$ Rule does not apply when the $\Delta\delta/J$ ratio becomes small, it is still possible to recognize these splitting patterns with the help of diagrams (such as those in Figures 5-2 through 5-6), and it is therefore possible to interpret the resonance.

There is an essential difference between the simple approach and that of quantum mechanics. In the simple model, the molecules are divided into groups and each group has a resonance at a different value of H_{ext}. In contrast, the quantum mechanical approach considers all the interacting magnetically active nuclei together and calculates the energy level differences and the probabilities of transition between energy levels. In the quantum mechanics model, all molecules are considered to be the same, but, according to the probabilities for different events to occur, a certain fraction will do one thing and another fraction will do another. In the AB system, for example, if $\Delta\delta/J$ is large, four transitions will have approximately the same probability. As $\Delta\delta/J$ decreases, the energies of these transitions and their probabilities change until at the A_2 limit only one transition is predicted to be observable.

Since, as was stated in section 3.3, coupling constants (J) are independent of H_{ext} while chemical shift differences ($\Delta\delta$) increase with H_{ext}, the $\Delta\delta/J$ ratio will be larger the larger H_{ext}. Thus distorted $N + 1$ Rule spectra will have a more nearly "first order" appearance the larger the magnetic field of the instrument used to obtain the spectrum. For example, suppose that a spectrum was obtained using a 60 MHz instrument and that it contained an ethyl resonance which looked like the one in Figure 5-6b; if the spectrum were to be redetermined on a 300 MHz instrument, the ethyl resonance would look like the one in Figure 5-6a.

5.2   THREE OR MORE COUPLED SETS OF NUCLEI

It is possible to express the change in splitting pattern from the $A_m X_n$ system, where the $N + 1$ Rule applies, through the $A_m B_n$ system, where it is necessary to use the methods of quantum mechanics to account for the splitting patterns, as a function of the $\Delta\delta/J$ ratio, if only two sets of coupled nuclei are involved. If, however, sets of magnetically active nuclei are present at three different chemical shifts (and magnetic equivalence is involved), the appearance of the spectrum depends upon three interset coupling constants (J_{AM}, J_{AX}, and J_{MX}) and two chemical shift differences (the third is determined by the other two), and it is impossible to present the possibilities in a systematic way as a function of a single parameter. The only simple thing that can be said is that the splitting pattern will be complex.

An example of such a system is that of acrylonitrile. While the $N + 1$ Rule would predict that the spectrum should show three pairs of doublets, as in the spectrum of p-chlorostyrene (Figure 4-11), the spectrum is complex and shows

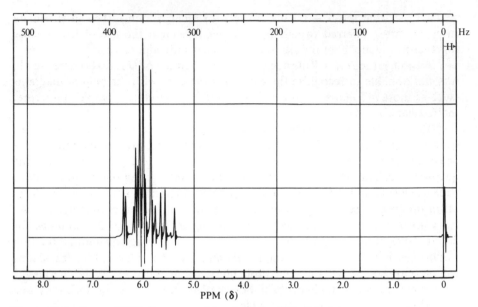

Figure 5-7   Proton NMR Spectrum of Acrylonitrile; CCl_4 Solution.

acrylonitrile

a total of fifteen lines (Figure 5-7). The reason is that in this molecule the chemical shift differences between the three protons are not large relative to the corresponding coupling constants. Acrylonitrile would be called an example of an *ABC* system.

When more nuclei are involved in three or more sets at different chemical shifts, the spectra are even more complex.

6 Complex Splitting Patterns: Magnetic Non-equivalence

In Chapter 4 the splitting patterns in the NMR spectra of several compounds were interpreted in a simple way, according to the $N + 1$ Rule. At that time, however, it was stated that two conditions must be met in order for the $N + 1$ Rule to apply. First, all coupling constants between members of two sets of magnetically active nuclei at different chemical shifts must be equal. Second, this one interset coupling constant, J, must be small relative to the chemical shift difference, $\Delta\delta$, between the two sets of magnetically active nuclei. In the preceding chapter we saw that if the second condition was not met, the splitting pattern generally had more lines than the $N + 1$ Rule could account for, and the relative intensities of the lines were not related to one another in any simple way. In this chapter we shall see that if the first condition is not met, complex splitting patterns will also be observed, even if the chemical shift differences are large.

So far, we have chosen only examples that satisfy the first condition. A simple molecule for which the protons do not satisfy this condition is 1-bromo-4-chlorobenzene. The two protons ortho to the bromine have the same chemical

1-bromo-4-chlorobenzene

shift, and the two protons ortho to the chlorine also have the same chemical shift; the chemical shifts of the two sets of protons are different. However, the interset coupling constants between the two magnetically active nuclei in each set are *not*

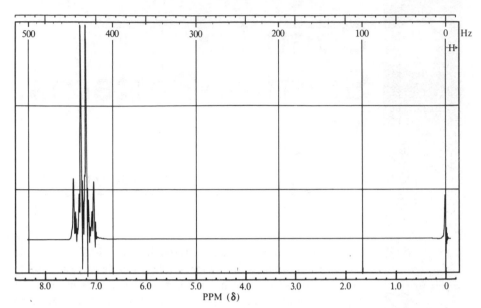

Figure 6-1 Proton NMR Spectrum of 1-Bromo-4-chlorobenzene; CCl_4 Solution.

all the same: for any proton in one set, there is one in the other set ortho to it and one in the other set para to it, and J_{ortho} is generally larger than J_{para}. The fact that there are two different interset coupling constants, J_{ortho} and J_{para}, means that first condition is not satisfied, and consequently the NMR spectrum of 1-bromo-4-chlorobenzene, which is shown in Figure 6-1, is complex and cannot be interpreted in terms of the $N + 1$ Rule.

It is often convenient to refer to the relationship between members of two sets of magnetically active nuclei at different chemical shifts in a brief way. The significant relationship for NMR spectroscopy is that of the equality or non-equality of the interset coupling constants, and the term *magnetic equivalence** is used to refer to sets of coupled magnetically active nuclei at two different chemical shifts for which all interset coupling constants are exactly equal. All previous examples, except the last (that of 1-bromo-4-chlorobenzene), have involved sets of magnetically equivalent nuclei, and the first prerequisite condition for the application of the $N + 1$ Rule could have been stated more briefly by saying that the sets of neighboring nuclei must be magnetically equivalent. In contrast, the two sets of protons in 1-bromo-4-chlorobenzene are said to be magnetically non-equivalent: *not* all of their interset coupling constants are equal.

---

* The term magnetic equivalence is used by different writers to mean several different things. However, since the question of whether or not the very useful $N + 1$ Rule can apply depends upon equality of interset coupling constants, we believe the term magnetic equivalence should be used to refer to this important condition.

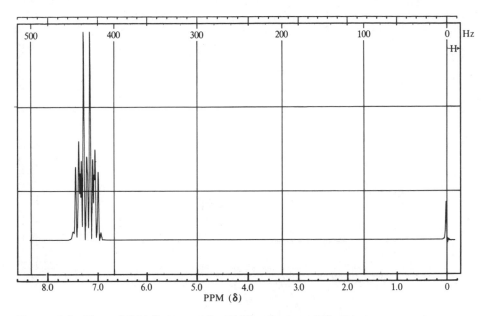

Figure 6-2 Proton NMR Spectrum of o-Dichlorobenzene; CCl₄ Solution.

Other examples of magnetic nonequivalence can be found in ortho di-substituted benzene derivatives where the two substituents are the same. In the case of 1,2-dichlorobenzene, J_{ortho} and J_{meta} relate members of the two sets of

magnetically active nuclei at different chemical shifts, and the spectrum (shown in Figure 6-2) is complex. Spin systems such as those of 1-bromo-4-chlorobenzene and 1,2-dichlorobenzene have often been referred to as $AA'XX'$ systems in which it is implied that J_{AX} is not equal to $J_{A'X}$ and therefore magnetic non-equivalence is involved.

In the case of a rigid molecule such as benzene, it is easy to tell whether coupling constants are necessarily equal to one another: if the geometrical relationships between pairs of magnetically active nuclei are exactly the same, the coupling constants must be identical. If the geometrical relationships between pairs of magnetically active nuclei are different, the coupling constants will usually be different although they might accidentally be the same. It is more difficult to decide whether interset coupling constants are equal or not (whether magnetic equivalence or magnetic nonequivalence is involved) with nonrigid molecules that can undergo conformational changes. For example, in 1-bromo-2-chloroethane, the two sets of protons—the two methylene groups—are

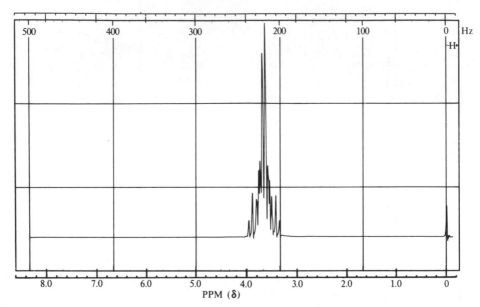

Figure 6-3 Proton NMR Spectrum of 1-Bromo-2-chloroethane; CCl₄ Solution.

magnetically nonequivalent (although this is not as obvious as in the case of 1-bromo-4-chlorobenzene), and the proton NMR spectrum (Figure 6-3) is complex.*

1-Bromo-2-chloroethane

So far in our interpretation of splitting patterns, we have considered only *interset* coupling constants—coupling constants between members of sets of magnetically active nuclei at different chemical shifts—and have never mentioned *intraset* coupling constants—coupling constants between magnetically active nuclei that have the same chemical shift. The reason is that when magnetic equivalence is involved, the appearance of the NMR spectrum is independent of all intraset coupling constants.

When magnetic nonequivalence is involved, however, as in the three examples of $AA'XX'$ systems presented in this chapter, the appearance of the NMR spectrum depends not only upon the difference in chemical shift between the two sets of magnetically active nuclei, $\Delta\delta$, but also upon the two different interset coupling constants, J_{AX} and $J_{A'X}$, *and* the two intraset coupling constants,

---

* A straightforward procedure by which one can determine whether or not magnetic equivalence is involved is described in the *Journal of Chemical Education*, vol. 51, p. 729, 1974.

$J_{AA'}$, and $J_{XX'}$. (In each of the three cases described above, $J_{AX} = J_{A'X'}$ and $J_{A'X} = J_{AX'}$ because of the symmetry of the molecule.) Since the appearance of the spectrum depends upon one chemical shift difference and four coupling constants, it is impossible to present the various ways in which the spectrum might appear as a function of a single parameter, as in the $A_m X_n$ systems. However, as you can see from Figures 6-1 through 6-3, the spectrum will always be symmetrical about its midpoint. This will also be true of any $A_m X_n$ system in which $m = n$, such as the AX system or the $A_2 X_2$ system (Figures 5-3 and 5-5).

Other systems in which magnetic nonequivalence is involved include mono-substituted benzene derivatives, such as acetophenone. Since the A and B pro-

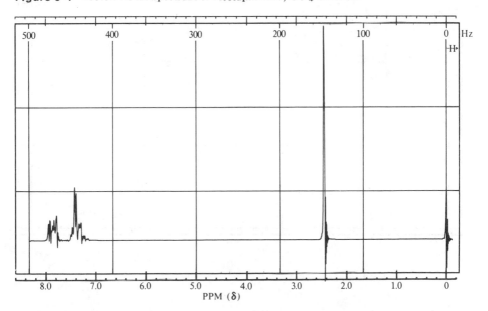

Acetophenone

tons are not magnetically equivalent, a complex resonance would be expected for the five aromatic protons. The spectrum (Figure 6-4) is in agreement with this expectation. The methyl protons, which make up an isolated A_3 system, appear as a singlet. However, in many monosubstituted benzene derivatives,

Figure 6-4   Proton NMR Spectrum of Acetophenone; CCl_4 Solution.

the presence of the substituent does not result in a significant difference in chemical shift between the ortho, meta, and para protons. When this is the case, the five protons make up a spin system that is very nearly an A_5 system in which the resonance should appear as a singlet and be independent of all coupling constants. An example illustrating this situation is that of toluene whose NMR spectrum shows a singlet for the aromatic protons as well as for the methyl

$$H_A \underset{H_B}{\overset{CH_3}{\diagdown}} H_{A'} \\ H_C \quad H_{B'}$$

toluene

protons (Figure 6-5). The difference in appearance of the resonance of the five aromatic protons of acetophenone and of toluene (Figures 6-4 and 6-5) can be explained by saying that the electron-withdrawing effect of the carbonyl group serves to deshield the protons ortho to it more than the ones meta and para to it thus spreading the ortho, meta, and para protons out over a range of chemical shifts.

Figure 6-5 Proton NMR Spectrum of Toluene; CCl_4 Solution.

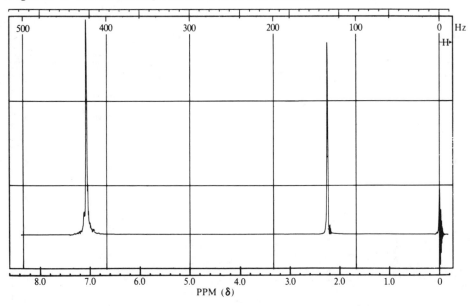

PROBLEMS

For each of the following compounds indicate which of the proton spin systems involve magnetic equivalence and which do not. Predict the appearance of the proton NMR spectrum of each compound. In the case of the resonance of a set of protons for which magnetic equivalence is not involved the prediction must be a "complex multiplet."

6-1.
$$CH_3-\overset{\overset{\displaystyle O}{\|}}{C}-O-CH_2CH_2-O-\overset{\overset{\displaystyle O}{\|}}{C}-CH_3$$

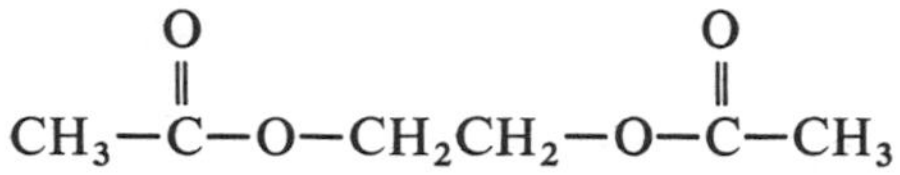

6-2.
$$CH_3-O-\overset{\overset{\displaystyle O}{\|}}{C}-CH_2CH_2-\overset{\overset{\displaystyle O}{\|}}{C}-O-CH_3$$

6-3.
$$CH_3-\overset{\overset{\displaystyle O}{\|}}{C}-O-CH_2CH_2-\overset{\overset{\displaystyle O}{\|}}{C}-O-CH_3$$

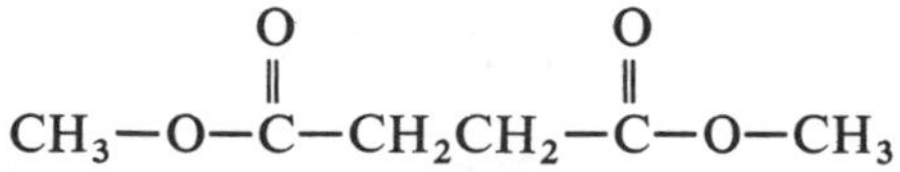

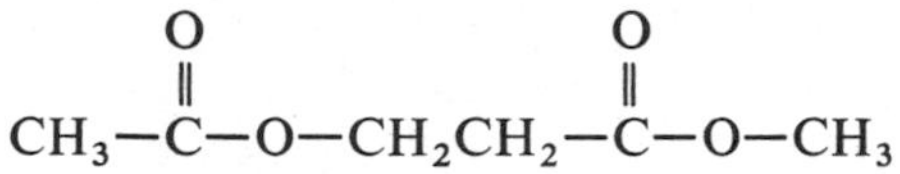

6-4.
7

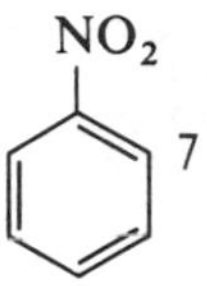

6-5.   ortho-dinitrobenzene
6-6.   meta-dinitrobenzene
6-7.   para-dinitrobenzene

6 8.
$$CH_3\ O-\overset{\overset{\displaystyle O}{\|}}{C}-CH_3$$

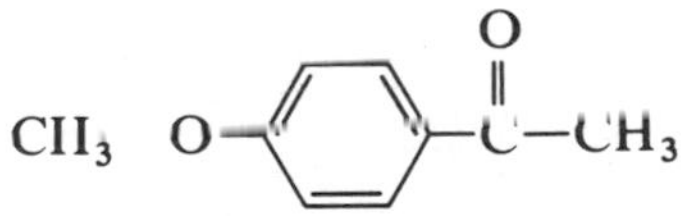

7 Interpretation of Proton NMR Spectra in Terms of Molecular Structure

In this chapter we will briefly consider some of the features of molecular structure that determine the degree of shielding of protons and the strength of coupling between protons. Then we will look at some more spectra of compounds of known structure in preparation for a consideration of how to approach the interpretation of the NMR spectrum of an unknown compound. Finally, we will mention some additional techniques that can be used as aids in the interpretation of NMR spectra.

7.1 DEPENDENCE OF CHEMICAL SHIFT UPON MOLECULAR STRUCTURE

In general, a proton on carbon is less shielded when there are strongly electron-withdrawing atoms or groups also bonded to that carbon atom. The more electron-withdrawing the group or the larger the number of such groups, the less the shielding. Thus the methylene protons of ethyl chloride (CH_3CH_2Cl) are less shielded than the methyl protons (Figure 4-10), and the methine proton 1,1,2-trichloroethane ($CHCl_2$—CH_2Cl) is less shielded than the methylene protons (Figure 4-5), Apparently a decrease in electron density in the vicinity of the proton results in less shielding. It is as if the action of the external magnetic field sets up a current which in turn produces a magnetic field in a direction opposing H_{ext}, thus serving to diminish the effect of H_{ext}. The lower the electron density about the proton, the smaller the induced current and the less the shielding.

Table 7-1   Chemical Shift—Molecular Structure Correlations for Protons on Carbon

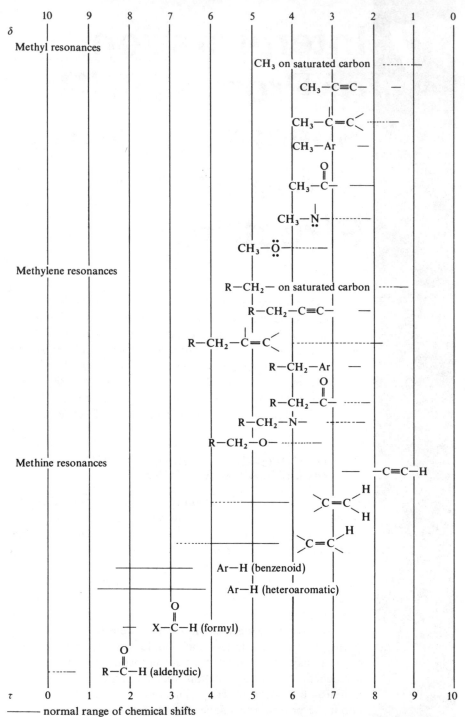

—— normal range of chemical shifts

······· range of chemical shifts when substituents are strongly electron withdrawing, either through inductive or resonance effects

Table 7-1 presents some observed correlations between chemical shift (shielding relative to the methyl protons of tetramethylsilane) and molecular structure. The first part of the table indicates the normal range of chemical shift for methyl groups in various structural environments. From this you can see that, in general, the more electronegative the atom or group to which the methyl is bonded the less shielded it is.

The middle part of Table 7-1 indicates the normal range of chemical shift for methylene groups in various structural environments. Comparing this part of the table with the first part shows that a methylene group such as $R-CH_2-$ is somewhat less shielded than a methyl group in the same structural environment. Apparently the alkyl group, R, has a deshielding effect relative to a hydrogen atom. If R is more electronegative than alkyl, the methylene group will be still less shielded. Table 3-1 presents more correlations between chemical shift and molecular structure for methylene groups of the type $X-CH_2-Y$.

The last part of Table 7-1 shows the normal range of chemical shifts of methine protons in various structural environments. Here you can see that a proton bonded to an aromatic ring is much less shielded than would be expected on the basis of electronegativity and inductive effects, and a special mechanism of deshielding is proposed to account for this. In any orientation of the aromatic ring with respect to the direction of the external magnetic field, H_{ext}, the π electrons will circulate in such a way as to produce a small magnetic field which will oppose the external field. This effect, however, will be largest when the plane of the ring is perpendicular to the direction of H_{ext}. The result is that the predominant shielding effect will be that which results from this particular orientation of the aromatic ring. Figure 7-1 shows that this means that the net effect of the induced magnetic lines of force resulting from the circulation of the π electrons will oppose H_{ext} inside the ring but will *augment* H_{ext} outside the ring. Since the aromatic protons are in the region of space where $H_{shielding}$ augments H_{ext}, they actually experience a deshielding effect. (H_{ext} can be less for resonance to occur.) Figure 7-2 indicates schematically that nuclei within or above or below an aromatic ring should be relatively shielded, whereas nuclei outside and more or less in the plane of the ring should be deshielded.

Figure 7-1   Induced Magnetic Lines of Force Resulting From Diamagnetic Ring Current in Benzene.

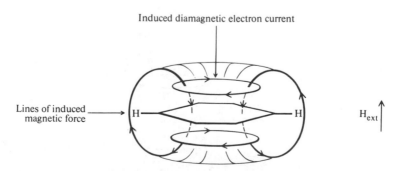

Induced diamagnetic electron current

Lines of induced magnetic force → H — — H H_{ext}

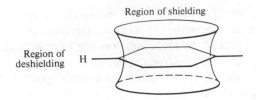

Figure 7-2   Magnetic Anisotropy of the Benzene Ring

A property which varies with direction is said to be *anisotropic*, and this type of directional dependence of shielding-deshielding is usually called *diamagnetic anisotropy*. Other π electronic systems such as C=O, C=C, and C≡C exhibit diamagnetic anisotropy; their regions of shielding and deshielding are indicated schematically in Figure 7-3.

The great deshielding of aldehydic and formyl hydrogens must be considered to be the result of both electron withdrawal by the carbonyl group and the effect of diamagnetic anisotropy. On the basis of electronegativity, acetylenic

Figure 7-3   Magnetic Anisotropy of the Carbonyl Group, the Carbon-Carbon Double Bond, and the Carbon-Carbon Triple Bond.

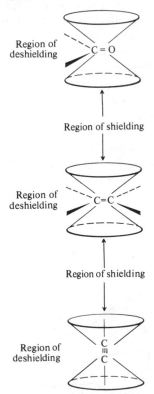

hydrogens would be expected to be less shielded than olefinic hydrogens (acetylene is far more acidic than ethylene); the fact that they are more shielded can be explained in terms of the effect of overcompensation due to diamagnetic anisotropy with the acetylenic proton in the relatively shielded region.

So far, we have only considered the expected chemical shifts for protons bonded to carbon. It is much more difficult to predict the positions of peaks due to protons on oxygen, nitrogen, or sulfur since they are relatively acidic and will also be involved in hydrogen bonding. Since the extent of hydrogen bonding is dependent upon concentration, solvent, and temperature, the position of the resonance of hydrogen bonded protons will be quite variable and will depend strongly upon the concentration of the sample, the solvent, and the temperature.

An interesting exception may be found when the hydrogen bonding is intramolecular (within the same molecule) rather than intermolecular (between different molecules). For example, acetylacetone exists partially in the enol form, and the chemical shift of the hydrogen bonded proton ($\delta = \sim 15$) is

keto   enol

acetylacetone

relatively insensitive to changes in concentration, solvent, and temperature.

In the case of the intramolecular hydrogen bond, the chemical shift of the acidic hydrogen is a measure of the stength of the bond. The enol form of acetylacetone has a strong hydrogen bond ($\delta = \sim 15$), while the bonds of o-hydroxyacetophenone ($\delta = \sim 12$) and o-hydroxybenzaldehyde ($\delta = \sim 11$) are somewhat weaker.

o-hydroxyacetophenone   o-hydroxybenzaldehyde

Table 7-2 presents some expected chemical shift ranges for protons bonded to oxygen, nitrogen, and sulfur.

Table 7-2   Chemical Shift—Molecular Structure Correlations for Protons on Oxygen, Nitrogen, and Sulfur

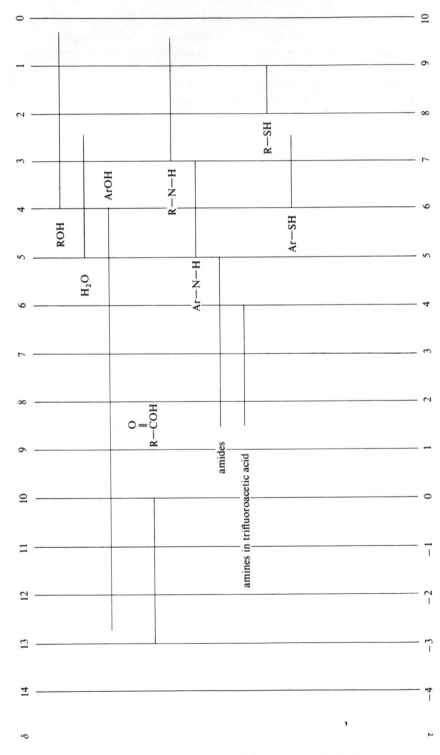

7.2 DEPENDENCE OF COUPLING CONSTANTS UPON MOLECULAR STRUCTURE

When discussing the dependence of coupling constants, J, upon molecular structure, it is important to distinguish between two types of molecules. The first is the conformationally mobile molecule that is rapidly changing from one conformation to another by rotating about single bonds. In the case of such molecules, average coupling constants will be involved.

The second type of molecule is the conformationally rigid one that cannot undergo rapid conformational isomerization, usually because of its cyclic structure. With such molecules, the coupling constants will correspond to a particular conformation or geometry. Of course, there are mixed systems in which a flexible side chain is connected to a rigid ring system.

In the conformationally mobile molecules, the average coupling constant, J, between aliphatic protons on adjacent carbon atoms is usually observed to be about 7 Hz; these protons are separated by three single bonds (H—C—C—H: $J = \sim 7$ Hz). This is the splitting that can be seen in Figures 4-5 through 4-10. Protons situated 1,3 to each other are separated by four single bonds and are rarely observed to be coupled to one another; coupling constants between protons separated by four single bonds are usually less than 0.5 Hz. (H—C—C—C—H: $J = \sim 0$). The coupling constant between aliphatic protons on the same carbon atom, separated by two single bonds, varies from zero to 30 Hz, depending upon the H—C—H bond angle (H—C—H: $J = \sim 0$ to ~ 30 Hz.). However, when these protons are magnetically equivalent, the appearance of the spectrum is independent of this coupling constant. In such cases the coupling constant cannot be determined from the spectrum. In predicting the NMR spectrum of a substance from its molecular structure, the effects of protons more distant than three single bonds may ordinarily be ruled out.

In the benzene ring, the coupling constant between ring protons decreases in the order ortho (6–10 Hz) to meta (2–3 Hz) to para (0–1 Hz). With olefins, however, the trans coupling constant is the largest (11–19 Hz), the cis smaller (5–11 Hz), and the geminal the smallest (0–3 Hz). This last example implies that the coupling effect is not transmitted through space but through the bonds between the atoms.

While the average coupling constant between protons on adjacent carbon atoms is 7 Hz, as determined from the NMR spectra of the freely rotating molecules of acyclic compounds, this coupling constant is strongly dependent upon the dihedral angle, as determined from the spectra of cyclic, conformationally rigid molecules.

Table 7-3 presents correlations between proton-proton coupling constants and molecular structure for some common structural features.

7.3 PROTON NMR SPECTRA OF COMPOUNDS OF KNOWN STRUCTURE

One of the best ways to become skilled in the interpretation of NMR spectra of substances of unknown structure is to become familiar with the spectra of

Table 7-3   Coupling Constant—Molecular Structure Correlations for Proton-Proton Coupling

		J_{ab}, Hz	
		Range	Typical values
$\underset{H_b}{\overset{H_a}{C}}$ (C with H_a, H_b)	(acyclic)	0–30	12–15
$H_a-C-C-H_b$	(free rotation)	6–8	7
$H_a-C-C-H_b$	(rigid: depends upon dihedral angle)	0–12	
$H_a-C-C-C-H_b$		0–1	0
$C=C$ with H_a, H_b (geminal)		0–3	0–2
$H_a\,C=C\,H_b$ (cis)	(acyclic)	5–11	10
$H_a\,C=C\,H_b$ (trans)		11–19	17
$C=C$ with H_a, $C-H_b$		4–10	7
$H_a\,C=C\,C-H_b$		0–3	2
$H_a\,C=C\,C-H_b$		0–3	1.5
$C=CH_a-CH_b=C$		9–13	10
$H_a-C-\overset{O}{C}-H_b$		1–3	2–3
$C=C\,\overset{O}{C}-H_b\,(H_a)$		5–8	6
$H_a-C-C\equiv C-H_b$		2–3	
$H_a-C-C\equiv C-C-H_b$		2–3	
benzene ring with H_a, H_b	ortho	6–10	9
	meta	2–3	3
	para	0–1	~0

substances of known structure and to understand why the spectra appear as they do. Proton NMR spectra of a number of compounds of known structure have been discussed in detail in earlier chapters. In this section, we will analyze the spectra of several more compounds of known structure. These compounds will be a little more representative of the variety of substances that one is likely to encounter in a first course in organic chemistry.

Ethyl Acetate

$$CH_3-\overset{\overset{\textstyle O}{\|}}{C}-O-CH_2CH_3$$

The spectrum of ethyl acetate (Figure 7-4) shows a sharp singlet and a clear ethyl resonance made up of a $1:3:3:1$ quartet and a $1:2:1$ triplet. The integral would show that the relative intensities of the quartet and the triplet are as 2 is to 3. and that the intensity of the singlet is equal to that of the triplet. The singlet corresponds to the methyl bonded to the $C=O$, and the ethyl resonance corresponds to the ethyl group bonded to the oxygen atom. Notice how the components of the triplet and quartet slope upwards or "point" toward each other. This pointing often serves as a valuable clue as to which multiplets belong to the same spin system.

Methyl Propionate

$$CH_3-O-\overset{\overset{\textstyle O}{\|}}{C}-CH_2CH_3$$

The spectrum of methyl propionate (Figure 7-5) is similar to that of its isomer ethyl acetate. It consists of a sharp singlet and a somewhat distorted ethyl resonance. In methyl propionate, however, the methyl is bonded to the oxygen atom and the ethyl group to the $C=O$ rather than the other way around as in ethyl acetate. This structural difference is clearly reflected in the difference in chemical shift of the methyl singlet in the two spectra: when the methyl group is bound to oxygen (methyl propionate) it is much less shielded than when bound to $C=O$ (ethyl acetate). Simiarly, the methylene group is much less shielded when bound to oxygen (ethyl acetate) than when bound to $C=O$ (methyl propionate). These differences are generally observed and are summarized in Table 7-1. Again the methylene quartet and methyl triplet point toward one another. Despite the considerable similarity between the splitting patterns of the two spectra it is easy to tell which corresponds to each isomer.

Vinyl Propionate

$$\underset{H}{\overset{H}{>}}C=C\underset{H}{\overset{O-\overset{\overset{\textstyle O}{\|}}{C}-CH_2CH_3}{}}$$

The spectrum of vinyl propionate (Figure 7-6) shows a slightly distorted ethyl resonance like that of methyl propionate, and a very clear, first-order,

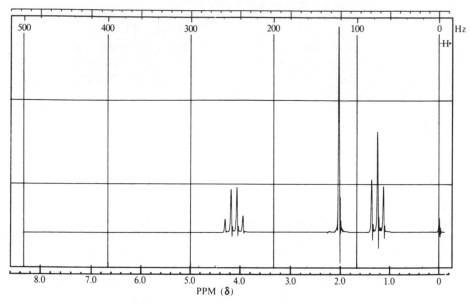

Figure 7-4   Proton NMR Spectrum of Ethyl Acetate; CDCl₃ Solution.

Figure 7-5   Proton NMR Spectrum of Methyl Propionate; CDCl₃ Solution.

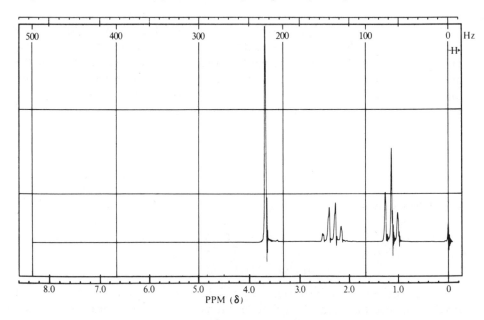

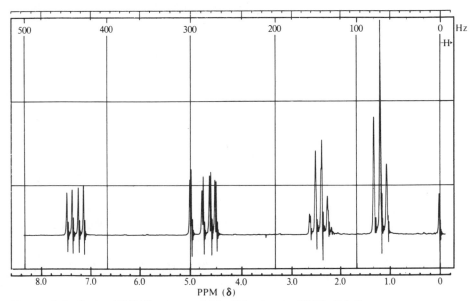

Figure 7-6   Proton NMR Spectrum of Vinyl Propionate; CDCl₃ Solution.

vinyl resonance made up of three pairs of doublets. The vinyl resonance of this compound is very similar to that of p-chlorostyrene (Figure 4-11). As previously indicated in Figure 4-12, the magnitude of the coupling of any one proton in a vinyl group to each of its neighbors is given by the spacing between lines 1 and 2, and 1 and 3 of the pair of doublets. Thus for p-chlorostyrene the proton whose resonance is centered at $\delta = 6.6$ is coupled to neighbors by $J = 18$ and $J = 12$, the proton whose resonance is centered at $\delta = 5.6$ is coupled to its neighbors by $J = 18$ and $J = 1$, and the proton whose resonance is centered at $\delta = 5.2$ is coupled to its neighbors by $J = 12$ and $J = 1$. Now, by referring to the correlations between molecular structure and coupling constants that are presented in Table 7-3, it is possible to assign the three pairs of doublets to the three vinyl protons: the resonance of H_A must appear at $\delta = 6.6$ since H_A would be expected to show splitting due to couplings of ~17 Hz and ~10 Hz, the resonance of H_M must appear at $\delta = 5.6$ since it would be expected to show splitting due to couplings of ~17 Hz and ~0–2 Hz, and the resonance of H_X must appear at $\delta = 5.2$ since it would be expected to show splitting due to couplings of ~10 Hz and ~0–2 Hz.

If a similar analysis is applied to the vinyl resonance of vinyl acetate, the resonance of the proton geminal to the oxygen is found to appear at $\delta = 7.3$, the resonance of the proton cis to the oxygen at $\delta = 4.85$, and the resonance of the proton trans to the oxygen at $\delta = 4.55$. It must be admitted that typical vinyl resonances are much more distorted than these and that they often appear to consist of less than 12 lines due to chance coincidences. Often, when the chemical shift differences are small, complex spectra will be observed; the spectrum of acrylonitrile (Figure 5-7) is an example of this.

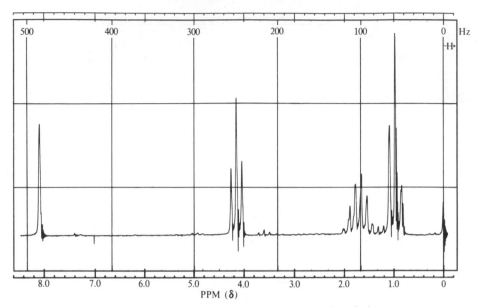

Figure 7-7   Proton NMR Spectrum of *n*-Propyl Formate; CDCl$_3$ Solution.

n-Propyl Formate

$$\underset{\displaystyle H-\overset{\displaystyle O}{\overset{\|}{C}}-O-CH_2-CH_2-CH_3}{}$$

The spectrum of *n*-propyl formate (Figure 7-7) can be interpreted by assigning the singlet at $\delta = 8.1$ to the formyl proton, the triplet at $\delta\ 4.1$ to the methylene bonded to oxygen, the triplet at $\delta = 1.0$ to the methyl group, and the multiplet centered at $\delta = 1.7$ to the middle methylene group. The methyl triplet is somewhat distorted since the chemical shift difference between the methyl protons and the neighboring methylene protons to which they are coupled is not very large. The small triplet centered at $\delta = 3.6$ is probably due to an impurity rather than to a spinning sideband (see section 9.1) since it is too intense and is at the wrong place for a spinning rate of 48 Hz.

Isopropyl Benzoate

The spectrum of isopropyl chloride was shown in Figure 4-9 to consist of a doublet for the methyl protons and a first order multiplet for the methine

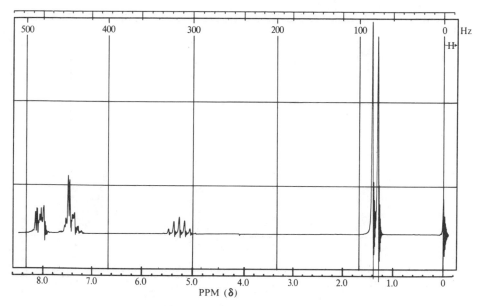

Figure 7-8   Proton NMR Spectrum of iso-Propyl Benzoate; $CDCl_3$ Solution.

proton. In the spectrum of isopropyl benzoate (Figure 7-8) the methine septet is centered at $\delta = 5.3$ and the methyl doublet at $\delta = 1.3$. At this spectrum amplitude, it is easy to miss the outer two peaks of the septet. Again, as with acetophenone (Figure 6-4), the two protons ortho to the electron-withdrawing carbonyl group are less shielded than the meta and para protons.

n-Butyl Chloride

$$Cl-CH_2CH_2CH_2CH_3$$

So far we have seen that the isolated methyl group always appears as a singlet and that the isolated ethyl group appears as a 1:3:3:1 quartet and a 1:2:1 triplet. The ethyl resonance can be somewhat distorted, however, unless the atom to which the methylene group is bonded is fairly electron-withdrawing so that the chemical shift difference between the methylene and the methyl groups is large. Examples involving the isolated n-propyl and isopropyl groups were shown in Figures 7-7 and 7-8. Again, however, the atom to which the alkyl group is bonded must be quite electronegative or else the splitting patterns will be much more distorted than in these two spectra.

We will now look at examples of the resonances of the four isomeric butyl groups. Figure 7-9 shows the spectrum of n-butyl chloride. The methylene group to which the electronegative chlorine is bonded gives a nice 1:2:1 triplet at $\delta = 3.55$, and the methyl group appears as a very distorted triplet at $\delta = 0.9$ since the protons of the neighboring methylene group to which the methyl protons are coupled are so similar in chemical shift. The resonance of the two inner methylene groups appears as a complex multiplet centered at $\delta = 1.7$.

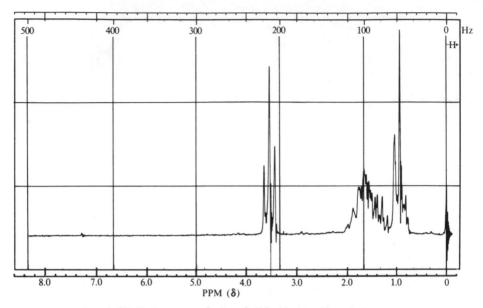

Figure 7-9 Proton NMR Spectrum of *n*-Butyl Chloride; $CDCl_3$ Solution.

Isobutyl Chloride

$$
\begin{array}{c}
\quad\quad CH_3 \\
\quad\quad | \\
Cl-CH_2-C-H \\
\quad\quad | \\
\quad\quad CH_3
\end{array}
$$

Figure 7-10 shows the spectrum of isobutyl chloride. The methylene protons appear as a 1 : 1 doublet at $\delta = 3.35$ due to coupling with their single neighbor, and the six methyl protons appear as a 1:1 doublet at $\delta = 1.0$ for the same reason. The methine proton appears as a weak, complex, multiplet at $\delta = 2$ due to slightly different couplings with its six and two neighbors.

sec-Butyl Chloride

$$
\begin{array}{c}
\quad\quad Cl \\
\quad\quad | \\
CH_3-C-CH_2CH_3 \\
\quad\quad | \\
\quad\quad H
\end{array}
$$

The spectrum of *sec*-butyl chloride is shown in Figure 7-11. The methine proton appears as a regular sextet at $\delta = 4.0$ due to essentially equal coupling to the methyl and methylene protons on the adjacent carbon atoms. The methyl group adjacent to the one methine proton appears as a 1 : 1 doublet at δ 1.5, and the methyl group adjacent to the two methylene protons appears as a distorted 1 : 2 : 1 triplet at $\delta = 1.0$. The multiplet centered at $\delta = 1.8$ is due to the methylene protons that are coupled to both the methine proton and the methyl group at $\delta = 1.0$.

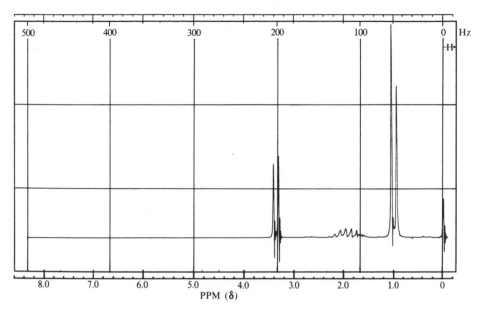

Figure 7-10 Proton NMR Spectrum of iso-Butyl Chloride; $CDCl_3$ Solution.

Figure 7-11 Proton NMR Spectrum of sec.-Butyl Chloride; $CDCl_3$ Solution.

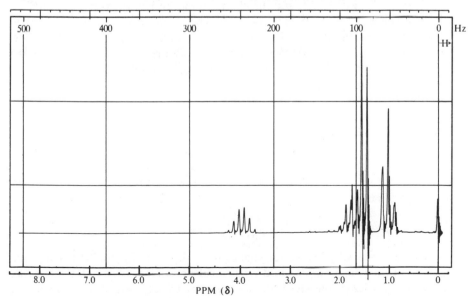

tert-Butyl Chloride

$$
\begin{array}{c}
CH_3 \\
| \\
Cl-C-CH_3 \\
| \\
CH_3
\end{array}
$$

The spectrum of *tert*-butyl chloride is shown in Figure 7-12. It consists of one line because the three methyl singlets must have the same chemical shift due to the symmetry of the molecule.

Again it is important to realize that when alkyl groups are bonded to less electron-withdrawing atoms or groups, their splitting patterns will be more distorted than those of the examples we have looked at.

p-Ethoxyacetanilide

Figure 7-13 shows the spectrum of *p*-ethoxyacetanilide, or phenacetin; this compound is used as an analgesic and antipyretic in APC tablets. The resonance centered at $\delta = 7.1$ is typical of unsymmetrically *p*-disubstituted benzene derivatives. The spectrum of 1-bromo-4-chlorobenzene is another example of this (Figure 6-1). The resonance of the isolated methyl in the acetyl group appears as a sharp singlet at $\delta = 2.1$, and the ethyl group bonded to oxygen gives a clear ethyl resonance at $\delta = 3.95$ and $\delta = 1.35$. The amide hydrogen gives a broad peak at $\delta = 8.3$. Protons bonded to nitrogen typically appear as rather wide, flat peaks and can be overlooked quite easily. Sometimes the position of the resonance of protons bonded to nitrogen can be determined more easily from the integral of the spectrum.

Ethyl p-Aminobenzoate

The spectrum of ethyl *p*-aminobenzoate is shown in Figure 7-14. This compound, benzocaine, is often used as a local anesthetic. Again, the resonance centered at $\delta = 7.2$ is consistent with an unsymmetrically *p*-disubstituted benzene

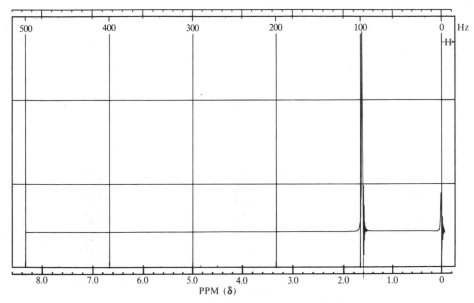

Figure 7-12   Proton NMR Spectrum of tert-Butyl Chloride; CDCl₃ Solution.

Figure 7-13   Proton NMR Spectrum of *p*-Ethoxyacetanilide; CDCl₃ Solution.

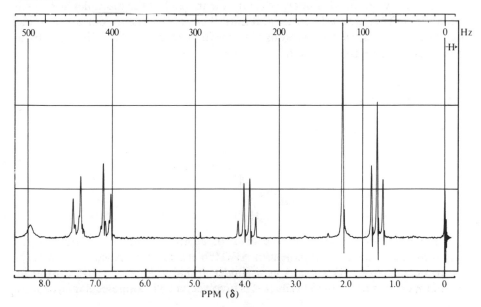

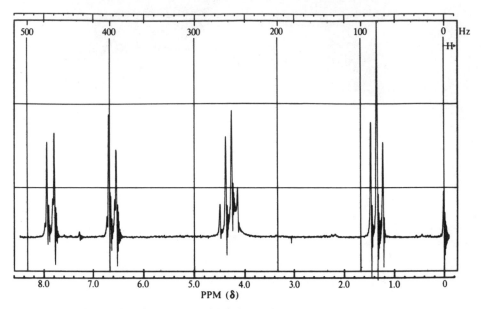

Figure 7-14   Proton NMR Spectrum of Ethyl p-Aminobenzoate; $CDCl_3$ Solution.

derivative, and the quartet and triplet are characteristic of an ethyl group bonded to an electronegative atom. The position of the resonance of the amino protons is not immediately apparent, but a closer look at the methylene quartet leads to the conclusion that the amino resonance must be present as a broad peak at $\delta = 4.2$ under the right side of the methylene quartet. Analysis of the integral of the spectrum confirms this interpretation: the integral of the multiplet at $\delta = 4.3$ equals that of the aromatic protons; it must therefore be due to four protons and not just the two methylene protons. The small peak at $\delta = 7.3$ is due to a trace of $CHCl_3$ in the $CDCl_3$ solvent.

Acetylsalicylic Acid

The spectrum of acetylsalicylic acid, or aspirin, is shown in Figure 7-15. The substance is another ingredient of APC tablets. The resonance of the methyl group bonded to C=O appears as a singlet at $\delta = 2.3$ The —OH proton in this compound is deshielded because it is involved in an intramolecular hydrogen

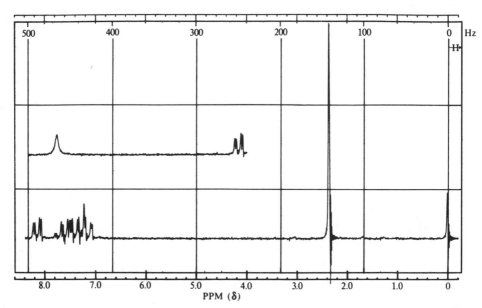

Figure 7-15   Proton NMR Spectrum of Acetylsalicylic Acid; CDCl₃ Solution; Offset = 48.

bond. The four aromatic protons each have a different chemical shift and their resonances appear as a complex multiplet between $\delta = 7.0$ and $\delta = 8.2$.

Methyl Salicylate

The spectrum of methyl salicylate, or oil of wintergreen, is shown in Figure 7-16. In this derivative of salicylic acid, the methyl singlet appears at $\delta = 3.9$, which is consistent with its being bonded to oxygen rather than to C=O as in salicylic acid, and the phenolic —OH proton appears as a sharp singlet at $\delta = 11.9$. The resonance of the aromatic protons of methyl salicylate is similar to that of the aromatic protons of acetylsalicylic acid. In both these unsymmetrically ortho-disubstituted benzene derivatives the resonance of the aromatic protons is unsymmetrical. This is in contrast to the resonance of o-dichlorobenzene (Figure 6-2) and other symmetrically ortho-disubstituted compounds for which the resonance of the aromatic protons will be symmetrical though complex.

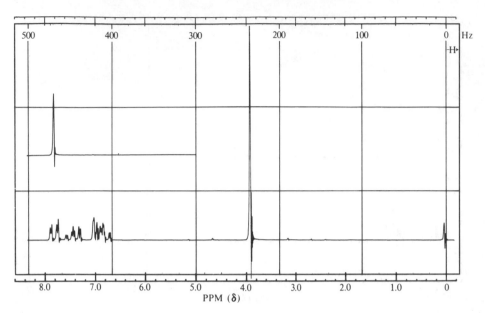

Figure 7-16 Proton NMR Spectrum of Methyl Salicylate; $CDCl_3$ Solution; Offset $= 3\delta$.

N,N-Diethyl-*m*-Toluamide

The spectrum of N,N-diethyl-*m*-toluamide, sold as an insect repellent under the name of "Off", is shown in Figure 7-17. The resonance for the aromatic methyl group appears as the expected sharp singlet at $\delta = 2.3$. However, while the quartet and triplet for the ethyl groups appear at their normal positions, their component peaks are unexpectedly broad. The reason for the broadening cannot be deduced without obtaining further spectra at different concentrations, solvents, and temperatures. Although, in principle, all four aromatic protons should experience different shielding and a complex resonance should be seen, the appearance of the aromatic resonance indicates that the actual differences in chemical shift must be very small. The situation is similar to that observed in the case of toluene (Figure 6-5) and must also obtain in the case of *p*-chlorostyrene (Figure 4-11). The small hump on the right side of the methylene quartet is a spinning sideband (see Section 9.1) as are also the small peaks at $\delta = 7.95$, 6.45, and 1.65.

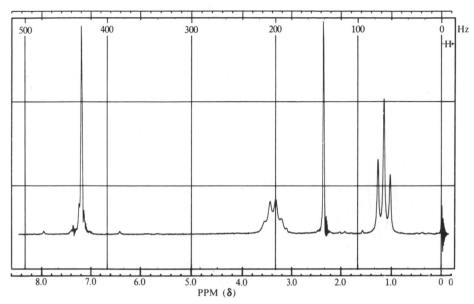

Figure 7-17   Proton NMR Spectrum of N, N-Diethyl-m-toluamide; CDCl₃ Solution.

2,4-Dichlorophenoxyacetic Acid

The spectrum of 2,4-dichlorophenoxyacetic acid, often called 2,4-D, is shown in Figure 7-18. The resonance of the —OH proton appears as a broadened singlet at $\delta = 10$, and the resonance of the methylene group appears as a sharp singlet at $\delta = 4.75$ that is in fair agreement with the value expected on the basis of the data of Table 3.1: $1.55 + 3.23 + 0.23 = 5.01$. The appearance of the resonances of the aromatic protons is similar to those of 2,4-dinitrochlorobenzene (Figure 4-15), another 1,2,4-trisubstituted benzene derivative. With the help of the information in Table 7-3 it is possible to determine which peaks correspond to each of the three aromatic protons. The proton in the 6 position must correspond to the widely spaced doublet at $\delta = 6.8$ since we would expect to see splitting due only to coupling with the proton ortho to it in the 5 position ($J = \sim 9$ Hz). The proton in the 3 position must correspond to the closely spaced doublet at $\delta = 7.4$ since we would expect to see splitting due only to coupling with the proton meta to it in the 5 position ($J = \sim 3$ Hz). The proton

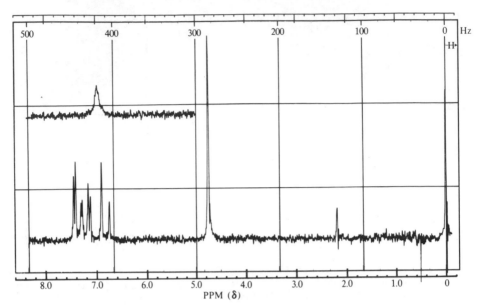

Figure 7-18 Proton NMR Spectrum of 2,4-Dichlorophenoxyacetic Acid; CDCl₃ Solution; Offset = 3δ.

in the 5 position must correspond to the pair of doublet centered at $\delta = 7.2$ since we would expect to see the resonance of this proton split by coupling to both of the other two protons ($J = \sim 9$ Hz and $J = \sim 3$ Hz).

The sharp singlet at $\delta = 2.2$ must be due to an impurity since the integral shows its intensity to be much less than that of the —OH resonance that corresponds to only one proton. A very likely possibility is acetone: its resonance appears at this chemical shift and it was used to clean the NMR sample tube. Since 2,4-dichlorophenoxyacetic acid was only slightly soluble, a dilute solution had to be used and the spectrum had to be scanned at a higher gain than the others, as you can see from the noisy baseline. It is under these conditions that impurities in solvents and sample tubes are most likely to be seen.

Vanillin

Figure 7-19 shows the spectrum of vanillin, the major flavor ingredient of vanilla extract. The resonance of the methyl group bonded to oxygen appears at $\delta = 3.95$, and the singlet due to the aldehyde proton appears at $\delta = 9.9$. The

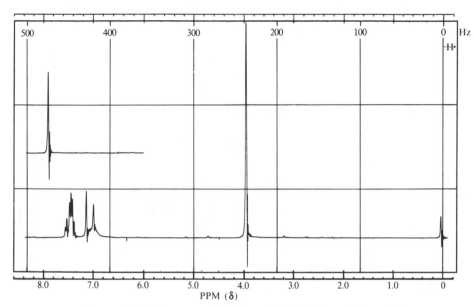

Figure 7-19   Proton NMR Spectrum of Vanillin; $CDCl_3$ Solution; Offset $= 2\delta$.

presence of a resonance at $\delta = 9.8$ to 10 is very characteristic of aldehydes. Since vanillin is also a 1,2,4-trisubstituted aromatic, one might hope that the resonance of the aromatic protons would be similar in appearance to those of 2,4-dichlorophenoxyacetic acid (Figure 7-18) and 2,4-dinitrochlorobenzene (Figure 4-15). Apparently the difference in chemical shift between the two protons para to one another is rather small giving the more complex multiplet centered at $\delta = 7.45$, and the —OH resonance lies at $\delta = 7.0$, under the right-hand member of the doublet, due to the proton para to the methoxy group. Evidently an intramolecular hydrogen bond involving an ethereal oxygen is rather weak since the —OH resonance of vanillin is at higher field than the —OH resonances of acetylsalicyclic acid and methyl salicylate (see Section 7-1).

Caffeine

The spectrum of caffeine, the third ingredient of APC tablets, is shown in Figure 7-20. For this substance, the three structurally different methyl groups bonded to nitrogen appear at slightly different chemical shifts, and the vinyl proton appears as a singlet at $\delta = 7.55$.

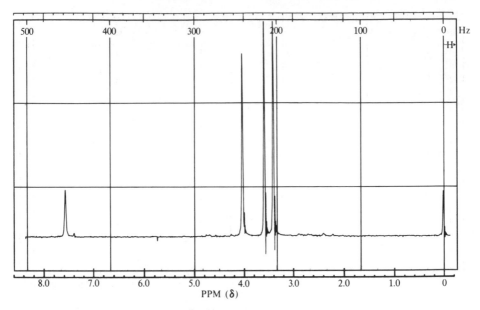

Figure 7-20 Proton NMR Spectrum of Caffeine; CDCl₃ Solution.

With this background we are now ready to consider the interpretation of the NMR spectra of two compounds of unknown structure.

7.4 INTERPRETATION OF THE PROTON NMR SPECTRUM OF AN UNKNOWN SUBSTANCE

In this section we will consider how one approaches the problem of determining the molecular structure of a substance from its NMR spectrum. Although there is usually information available in addition to the NMR spectrum, we will start by trying to obtain as much information as possible from the NMR spectrum alone. If the molecular formula is known as well, it is possible, in a favorable case, to determine with complete certainty the molecular structure of the unknown substance and to do this without comparing the spectrum of the unknown to the spectrum of an authentic sample of the substance. A similar identification could rarely be made using only the infrared or the ultraviolet spectrum.

The general approach to the determination of the molecular structure of a substance from its NMR spectrum is to consider each of the three aspects of the spectrum described in Chapter 3: the chemical shift, the integral, and the splitting patterns. From the number of resonances at different chemical shifts, you can tell how many sets of protons there are in different chemical environments in the molecule. From the integral, you can tell the relative number of protons in each set, and from the splitting pattern, you can get information as to the structural and geometrical relationships among the protons. From the correlations between chemical shift and molecular structure, and between coupling constants and molecular structure, a structure of the molecular fragments responsible for the various spectral features can be deduced and the fragments can then be put together to satisfy valence requirements and any other information that is available about the compound.

While so far we have emphasized the presence of peaks at certain chemical shifts, the absence of peaks in certain portions of the spectrum usually allows whole classes of compounds to be ruled out. For example, the absence of absorption above $\delta = 10$ rules out carboxylic acids; the absence of absorption at $\delta = 10$ rules out aldehydes; and the absence of absorption between $\delta = 6$ and 9 essentially rules out aromatics. If no peak appears higher than $\delta = 4$, other than ones attributable to carboxylic acid or aldehydic protons, the compound is almost certainly a saturated aliphatic.

As an example, consider the spectrum shown in Figure 7-21. Although this spectrum is not nearly as nice looking as the ones we have considered so far, it still contains a lot of information. Since the entire spectrum appears between $\delta = 0.8$ and $\delta = 3.8$, the substance can contain no olefinic nor aromatic protons. The highly distorted $1 : 2 : 1$ triplet centered at $\delta = 0.8$ is characteristic of a methyl group that is adjacent to a methylene group and at the end of a moderately long aliphatic side chain. The distorted $1 : 2 : 1$ triplet centered at $\delta = 3.6$ must correspond to two protons on the carbon bearing the functional group split, most likely, by the protons of a second methylene group at the next carbon atom. This triplet must correspond to two protons because it cannot correspond to three (the carbon bearing these protons must have at least two other groups

Figure 7-21   Proton NMR Spectrum of 1-Octanol; CDCl₃ Solution; trace of HCl Added.

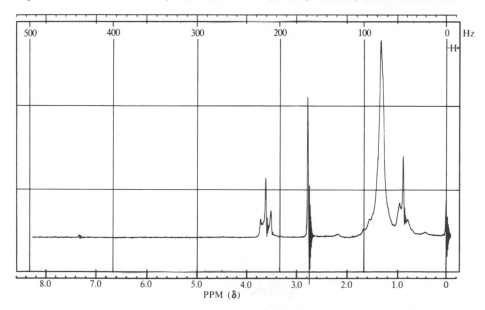

bonded to it: the functional group and the rest of the molecule), and it cannot correspond to only one (there would then have to be a second chain end and there is no evidence for another terminal methyl group in the spectrum). Thus the partial structures

$$X—CH_2—CH_2— \quad \text{and} \quad —CH_2—CH_3$$

have been established, and

$$\begin{array}{c} H \\ | \\ X—C— \\ | \end{array}$$

has been ruled out. A structure such as

$$X—CH_2—(CH_2)_n—CH_3$$

incorporates both these structural features and could also account for the broad resonance centered at $\delta = 1.3$ as the resonance of the n methylene groups that would all be very similar in chemical shift. The functional group X must account for the sharp singlet at $\delta = 2.8$. Two questions remain: what is n and what is X?

If we accept that the integral of the triplet at $\delta = 3.6$ corresponds to two protons, then the integral between $\delta = 2.4$ and 0.1 corresponds to 15.5 protons (Figure 7-22). Subtracting three for the methyl group, we are left with 12.5, and

Figure 7-22 Integral of Spectrum Shown in Figure 7-21.

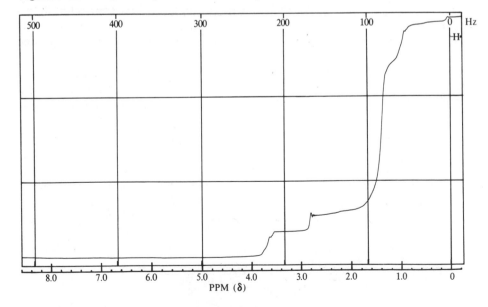

since the number of protons in the n methylene groups must be even, 12 is the best estimate; n must be then 6. The unknown appears to be a 1-octane derivative, $X-CH_2CH_2CH_2CH_2CH_2CH_2CH_2CH_3$, in which X must be able to account for the one proton singlet at $\delta = 2.8$.

It is more reasonable to propose that $X = -OH$ than aldehyde or carboxyl, for two reasons. The first is that a chemical shift of $\delta = 2.8$ is quite inconsistent with the other two possibilities. The second is that $-CH_2-R$ adjacent to oxygen would be expected to appear near $\delta = 3.6$, while $-CH_2-R$ adjacent to $C=O$ would be expected to appear near $\delta = 2.4$. The infrared spectrum, of course, could answer this question as well. Thus the spectrum is seen to be consistent with the structure 1-octanol, $HO-CH_2CH_2CH_2CH_2CH_2CH_2CH_2CH_3$.

Although the $-OH$ proton is only three bonds away from its methylene neighbor, it appears unsplit. This is because the rate of exchange of $-OH$ protons among alcohol molecules (intermolecular exchange) is fast and the contribution of the neighboring methylene protons to H_{ext} for the $-OH$ proton is averaged to zero for all $-OH$ protons. The methylene protons on the carbon bearing the $-OH$ group are likewise unsplit by the $-OH$ protons for the same reason. In fact, a trace of acid was added to the sample to ensure that the $H-O-CH_2-$ coupling was averaged to zero by sufficiently rapid acid-catalyzed intermolecular exchange.

The presence of hydroxyl, amino, carboxyl, or other easily exchanged protons can be determined or confirmed in another way. When the spectrum has been run in a solvent such as $CDCl_3$ or CCl_4, it can be rerun after adding a drop or two of D_2O, shaking thoroughly, and allowing the water to rise to the top. Exchangeable protons will be extensively replaced by deuterium and will not show up when the spectrum is rerun because they will be in the water layer floating above the sensitive volume of the spectrometer detector. When this is done to the sample of 1-octanol used to obtain Figure 7-21, the spectrum shown in Figure 7-23 is obtained. The peak at $\delta = 2.8$ has essentially disappeared. The small new peak near $\delta = 4.6$ is due to the protons in HOD dissolved or suspended in the sample solution.

As a final example, consider the spectrum shown in Figure 7-24. Again, it is not as nice a spectrum as those we have looked at earlier, but it still can yield much structural information. First, the compound contains no aromatic protons: the splitting pattern of the small multiplet of relative area one at $\delta = 6.8$ is much more characteristic of an olefinic proton than of an aromatic proton. Second, any methyl groups in the molecule must be bonded to unsaturated carbon: methyl groups on saturated carbon would appear (split, unless tert-butyl) near $\delta = 1$, and methyl groups on O, N, or $C=O$ would appear as sharp singlets at a chemical shift greater than two. The slightly split peak at $\delta = 1.8$ is consistent with methyl on unsaturated carbon, with the splitting due to coupling to olefinic protons.

If one next assumes that the multiplet of relative area two at $\delta = 4.8$ is also due to olefinic protons, the integral (Figure 7-25) indicates that the ratio of olefinic protons to aliphatic protons is 3 to 11, for a total of 14. If the compound

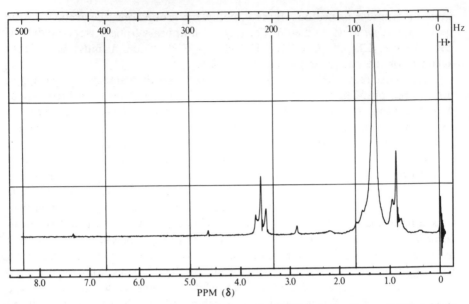

Figure 7-23 Proton NMR Spectrum of 1-Octanol; CDCl₃ Solution; trace of HCl Added; D₂O Added.

Figure 7-24 Proton NMR Spectrum of R-(−)-Carvone; CDCl₃ Solution.

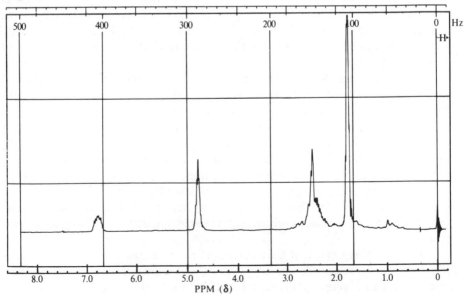

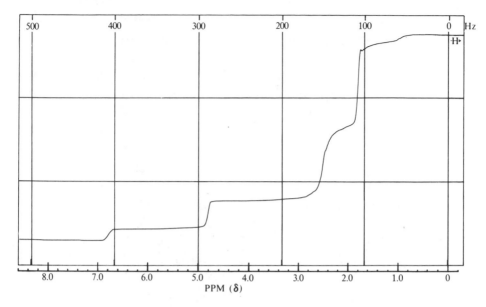

Figure 7-25 Integral of Spectrum Shown in Figure 7–24.

contains only carbon, hydrogen, and oxygen, (or an even number of nitrogen atoms), the total number of protons must be even. If the resonance at $\delta = 1.8$ is due to methyl protons, it must be equivalent to 3, 6, or 9 protons; the integral is most consistent with 6. To summarize, the spectrum is consistent with the presence of three olefinic protons, two methyl groups bonded to C=C, and five other relatively deshielded aliphatic protons. The sample was actually R-(−)-carvone.

PROBLEMS

7.1. Describe how you would distinguish the members of the following pairs of structural isomers or stereoisomers by means of their proton NMR spectra. (Predict the appearance of the proton NMR spectrum of each isomer and then point out the differences.)

a. $N\equiv C-CH_2CH_2-C\equiv N$ and $CH_3-\overset{\overset{\displaystyle C\equiv N}{|}}{\underset{\underset{\displaystyle C\equiv N}{|}}{C}}-H$

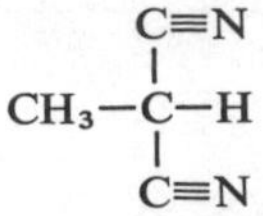

b. 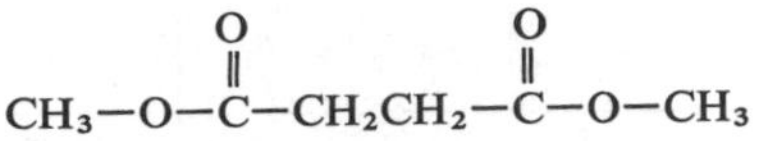 $CH_3-O-\overset{\overset{\displaystyle O}{\|}}{C}-CH_2CH_2-\overset{\overset{\displaystyle O}{\|}}{C}-O-CH_3$ and $CH_3-\overset{\overset{\displaystyle O}{\|}}{C}-O-CH_2CH_2-O-\overset{\overset{\displaystyle O}{\|}}{C}-CH_3$

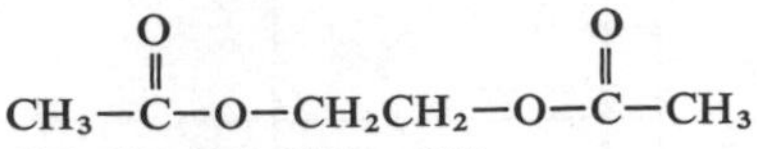

c. $CH_3CH_2-O-CH_2CH_3$ and $CH_3CH_2CH_2CH_2-OH$

d. $Cl-CH_2-CH_2-Br$ and $CH_3-\overset{\overset{\displaystyle Br}{|}}{\underset{\underset{\displaystyle Cl}{|}}{C}}-H$

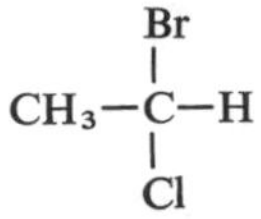

e. $CH_3-CH_2-CH_2-Cl$ and $CH_3-\overset{\overset{\displaystyle Cl}{|}}{\underset{\underset{\displaystyle H}{|}}{C}}-CH_3$

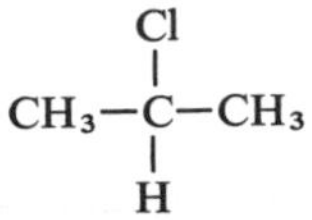

f. 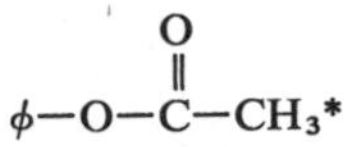 $\phi-O-\overset{\overset{\displaystyle O}{\|}}{C}-CH_3$*   and $\phi-\overset{\overset{\displaystyle O}{\|}}{C}-O-CH_3$

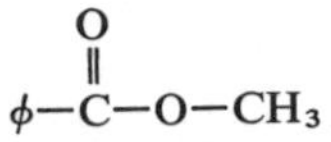

g. 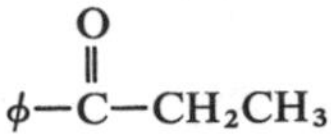 $\phi-\overset{\overset{\displaystyle O}{\|}}{C}-CH_2CH_3$ and $\phi-CH_2-\overset{\overset{\displaystyle O}{\|}}{C}-CH_3$

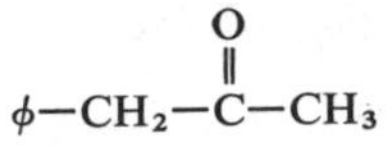

h. 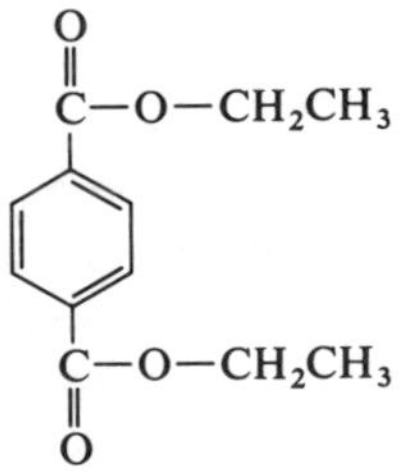
and

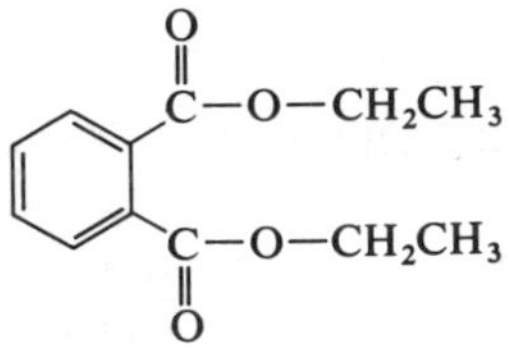

i. 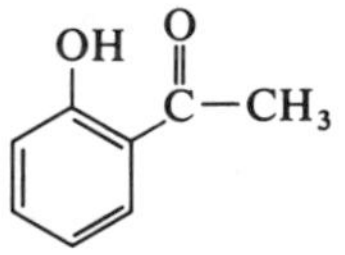
and

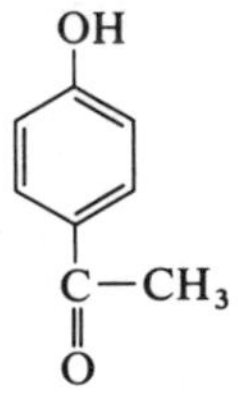

j. 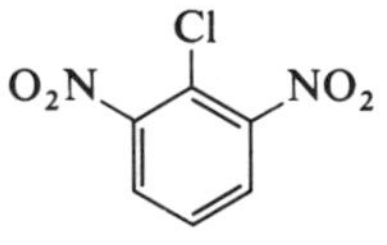
and

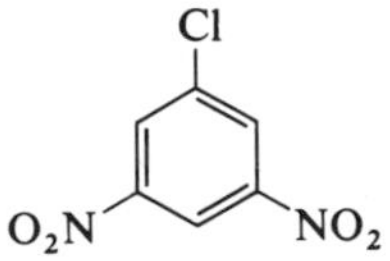

* ϕ stands for 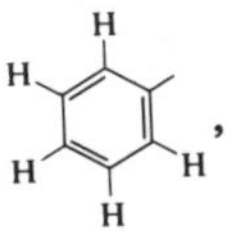 , the phenyl radical.

k.   and

l.   and   N≡C—CH₂CH₂—C≡N

m.   and

n.   and

o.   and

7.2. Describe how you would distinguish the members of the following sets of structural isomers by means of their proton NMR spectra. (Predict the appearance of the proton NMR spectrum of each isomer and then point out the differences.)

a. The three isomeric dichlorobenzenes.
b. The three isomeric trichlorobenzenes.
c. The isomers of molecular formula C_4H_9Br.
d. The isomers of molecular formula C_3H_8O.
e. The isomers of molecular formula C_3H_4.

7.3. Figure 7-26 shows the proton NMR spectrum of a substance of molecular formula C_2H_4O. Propose a structural formula for this substance.

7.4. Figure 7-27 shows the proton NMR spectrum of a substance of molecular formula C_3H_3Br. Propose a structural formula for this substance.

7.5. Figure 7-28 shows the proton NMR spectrum of a substance of molecular formula C_5H_8. Propose a structural formula for this substance.

7.6. Figures 7-29a, 7-29b, and 7-29c show the proton NMR spectra of three isomers of molecular formula C_4H_8O. Propose a structural formula for each isomer.

7.7. Figures 7-30a, 7-30b, and 7-30c show the proton NMR spectra of three isomers of molecular formula C_4H_6O. Propose a structural formula for each isomer.

7.8. Figure 7-31 shows the proton NMR spectrum of a substance of molecular formula $C_6H_{14}O_2$. Propose a structural formula for this substance.

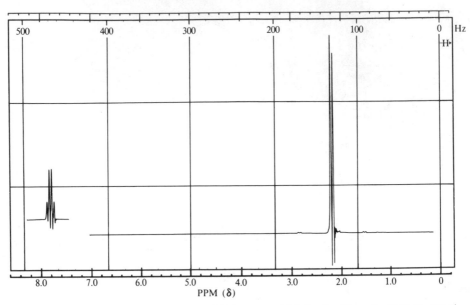

Figure 7-26 Proton NMR Spectrum of Substance of Molecular Formula C_2H_4O; Neat Liquid; Offset$=2\delta$.

Figure 7-27 Proton NMR Spectrum of Substance of Molecular Formula C_3H_3Br; CCl_4 Solution.

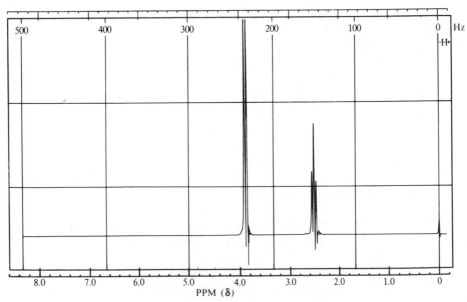

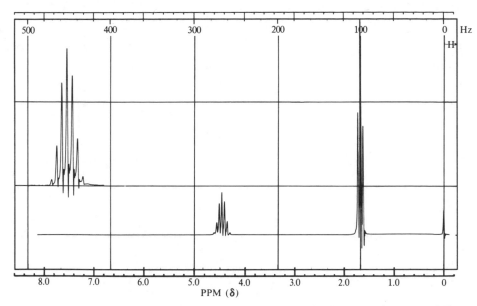

Figure 7-28 Proton NMR Spectrum of Substance of Molecular Formula C₅H₈; CCl₄ Solution. Inset shows an enlargement of the resonance at δ = 4.5.

Figure 7-29a Proton NMR Spectrum of Substance of Molecular Formula C₄H₈O; CCl₄ Solution

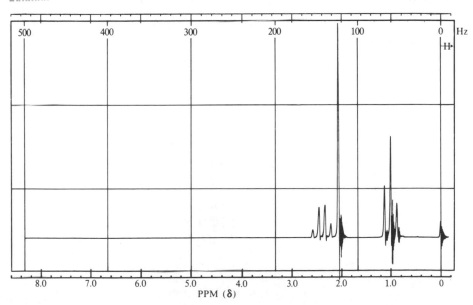

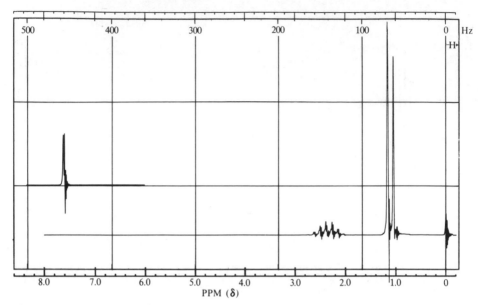

Figure 7-29b Proton NMR Spectrum of Substance of Molecular Formula C_4H_8O; CCl_4 Solution.   Offset $= 2\delta$.

Figure 7-29c Proton NMR Spectrum of Substance of Molecular Formula C_4H_8O; CCl_4 Solution.

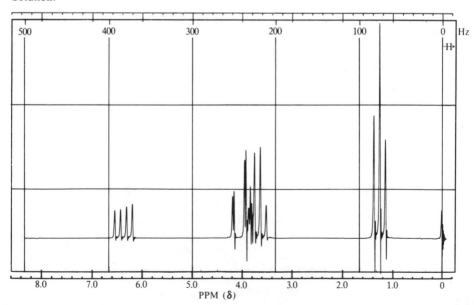

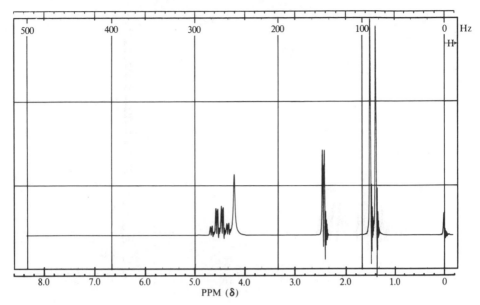

Figure 7-30a   Proton NMR Spectrum of Substance of Molecular Formula C_4H_6O; CCl_4 Solution.

Figure 7-30b   Proton NMR Spectrum of Substance of Molecular Formula C_4H_6O; CCl_4 Solution.

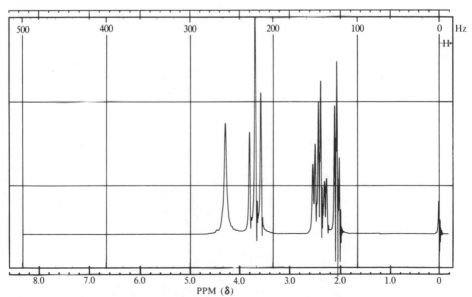

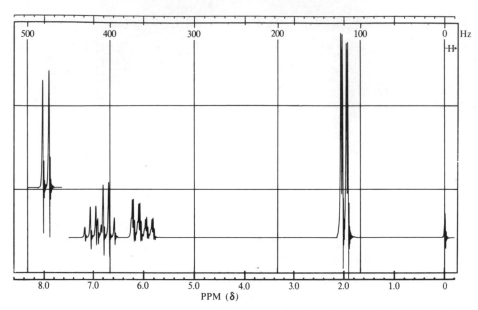

Figure 7-30c   Proton NMR Spectrum of Substance of Molecular Formula C_4H_6O; CCl_4 Solution. Offset $= 2\delta$.

Figure 7-31   Proton NMR Spectrum of Substance of Molecular Formula $C_6H_{14}O_2$; CCl_4 Solution.

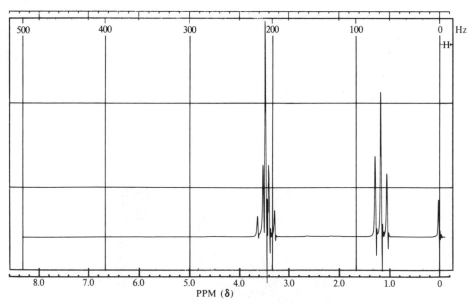

7.9. Figure 7-32 shows the proton NMR spectrum of a substance of molecular formula $C_7H_{16}O_4$. Propose a structural formula for this substance.

7.10. Figure 7-33 shows the proton NMR spectrum of a substance of molecular formula $C_{11}H_{20}O_4$. Propose a structural formula for this substance.

7.11. According to a procedure described in *Organic Syntheses*, α-chloroanisole can be prepared by treating a boiling solution of anisole in dichloromethane with sulfuryl chloride:

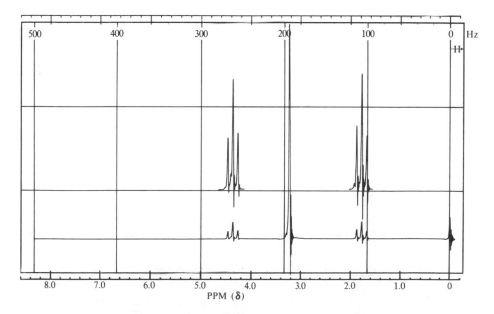

Since the product of the reaction failed to give a precipitate when treated with silver nitrate in ethanol, the proton NMR spectrum was determined. Figure 7-34 shows the spectrum of the product actually formed in the reaction. What was the actual product? (*J. Org. Chem.*, vol. 33, p. 3335, 1968).

7.12. Figure 7-35 shows the proton NMR spectrum of a substance of molecular formula $C_{12}H_{14}O_4$. Propose a structural formula for this substance.

7.13. Figure 7-36 shows the proton NMR spectrum of a substance of molecular formula $C_8H_6O_3$. Propose a structural formula for this substance.

Figure 7-32   Proton NMR Spectrum of Substance of Molecular Formula $C_7H_{16}O_4$; CCl_4 Solution.

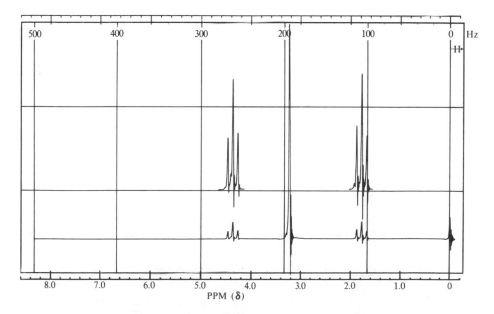

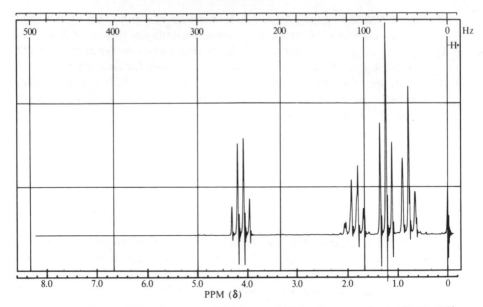

Figure 7-33 Proton NMR Spectrum of Substance of Molecular Formula $C_{11}H_{20}O_4$;CCl_4 Solution.

Figure 7-34 Proton NMR Spectrum and Integral of Substance Formed Upon Chlorination of Anisole; CCl_4 Solution.

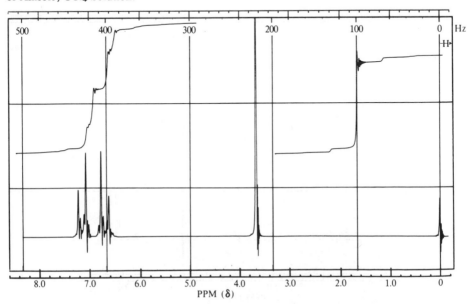

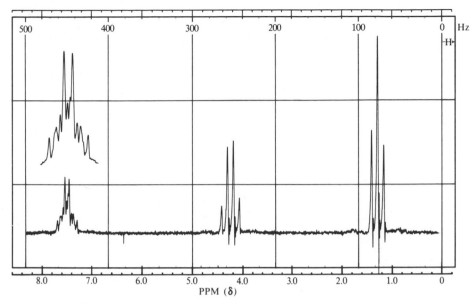

Figure 7-35   Proton NMR Spectrum of Substance of Molecular Formula $C_{12}H_{14}O_4$; CCl_4 Solution.

Figure 7-36   Proton NMR Spectrum of Substance of Molecular Formula $C_8H_6O_3$; CCl_4 Solution; Offset = 2δ.

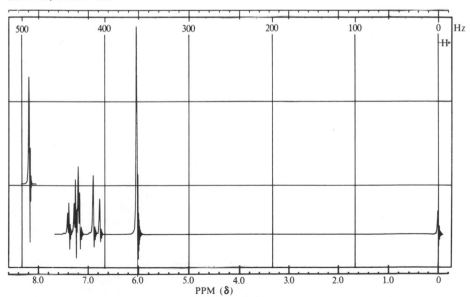

8 Preparation of the Sample

This chapter is concerned with the practical aspects of preparing suitable samples for NMR analysis. The topics that will be considered in the next sections include the amount and concentration of the sample required, the nature of the solvent, the type of container for the sample (the sample tube), and the use of reference standards.

8.1 SAMPLE

Amount

Thirty to 40 milligrams is the amount of the average organic compound needed to obtain a good NMR spectrum. For high resolution NMR spectrometry, the sample to be studied normally must be present as a liquid or a solution. Gases are usually studied in solution since otherwise they must be sealed under many atmospheres pressure in carefully annealed thick-walled glass tubing in order to obtain a sufficiently concentrated sample. Solids cannot be directly studied by high resolution NMR spectroscopy since intermolecular forces result in extremely broad lines, and a knowledge of crystal structure is required for interpreting such "broad line" NMR spectra. For this reason, solids must be dissolved in a solvent for use in high resolution NMR spectroscopy. The material to be studied can range from an analytically pure sample to a tarry distillation residue.

Although it is very convenient to determine the NMR spectrum of a liquid without using a solvent (using the neat liquid), there are two reasons for determining the spectra of liquids as well as solids as a solution. The first is that the liquid may be too viscous. If the viscosity is too high, certain intermolecular interactions will not be averaged to zero by molecular motion, and relatively broad peaks will be observed. Determining the spectrum of the liquid as a solution in a non-viscous solvent can eliminate this problem. The second reason is that chemical shift differences from tetramethylsilane (TMS) or any other reference standard can be strongly dependent upon both the nature of the solvent and the concentration. Thus if chemical shifts are to be compared with confidence, the comparisons must be made between spectra determined while using samples in dilute solution in the same solvent. The differences in chemical shifts determined with the neat liquid (or a concentrated solution) and those determined with a dilute solution are most likely to be large if the sample contains an aromatic ring. They can be accurately estimated, of course, only by actually determining spectra at different concentrations. The advantage of using a neat liquid or a concentrated solution is that weak peaks or impurities are more easily observed.

At a sufficiently low concentration, the peaks of the spectrum will be indistinguishable from the baseline noise of the NMR spectrometer. For both solids and liquids, the lowest useful concentration depends both upon the nature of the compound and upon the sensitivity of the NMR spectrometer. If you want to see the resonance of one proton that is split into a multiplet, the necessary sample concentration will be considerably larger than that needed to see a singlet due to several protons at the same chemical shift. Also, some NMR spectrometers are more sensitive than others; with a standard substance at a certain concentration, some NMR spectrometers produce a larger signal relative to the baseline noise than others. A common standard for comparison of proton NMR spectrometers is a 1 percent solution of ethylbenzene ($\phi-CH_2CH_3$) in carbon tetrachloride. The sensitivity is expressed as the ratio of the height of the tallest peak of the methylene quartet to the root-mean-square baseline noise (the peak-to-peak baseline noise divided by 2.4). This estimate of sensitivity—the signal-to-noise ratio, or S/N—is illustrated in Figure 8-1.

Dilute Samples

With very dilute samples, one generally loses resolution since the higher rf power needed for the best S/N ratio leads to some sample saturation and line broadening (see Section 9.1). The greater damping of the highly amplified output signal that may be desired in order to gain a reasonable S/N ratio will also broaden the spectral lines. With dilute samples, the accuracy of the integral is also lost. With a concentrated sample, a careful integration can yield proton ratios to within ± 1 percent; with a dilute sample, a 10 percent accuracy in proton ratios is considered acceptable. A usable spectrum can be obtained for a sample which will not yield a usable integral. Finally, a dilute sample requires greater care since slower scan speeds are necessary to obtain an adequate S/N ratio, and it is more difficult to avoid saturation. Several scans may be necessary in order to separate true signals from accidental noise.

Poorly Resolved Spectra

Certain compounds do not yield well resolved spectra. These include rigid poly-cyclic molecules such as bicycloheptane and steroid derivatives. One reason is that the chemical shift differences between ring protons are small and the small

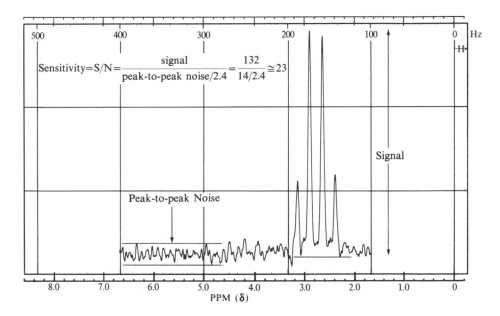

Figure 8-1   Determination of the Sensitivity of an NMR Spectrometer from the Resonance of the Methylene Quartet of a 1% Solution of Ethylbenzene.

$\Delta\delta/J$ ratios lead to more lines. The result is that the many closely spaced lines of the spectrum are not resolved and broad bands are seen. This same type of poorly resolved spectrum is also observed with long chain aliphatic compounds. The spectrum of 1 octanol, without added acid, is an example (Figure 8-2). Other spectra of 1-octanol were discussed in section 7.4.

Paramagnetic Impurities

Occasionally a particular sample will not yield a good spectrum. One cause of this may be the presence of paramagnetic impurities (impurities with unpaired electrons, such as iron or copper compounds). For example, several oxygenated aromatic compounds, benzoquinones, naphthoquinones, etc., gave improved NMR spectra when the samples used for the spectra had been sublimed. Apparently trace amounts of paramagnetic materials present with the compound after its preparation served to broaden the spectral lines, and these were left behind by sublimation of the sample. If a compound gives a poor spectrum with an instrument functioning well either with other samples or with the standard samples, you should attempt to purify it with respect to metal ions. Oximes, orthoquinones, β-diketones and other potential chelating agents can be quite troublesome in this respect. Organic salts normally give good NMR spectra, but sometimes metal ions present in the acid or base added to produce the salt result in a degraded spectrum.

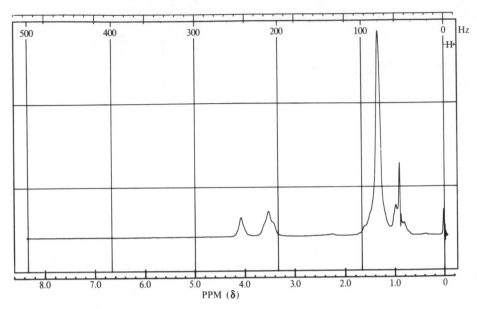

Figure 8-2   Proton NMR Spectrum of 1-Octanol; CCl₄ Solution; No Acid Added.

Ferromagnetic Impurities

Poor resolution is occasionally due to the presence of suspended ferromagnetic particles such as iron filings. These may be removed by touching the bottom of the sample tube to a powerful permanent magnet and then moving the tube so the point of contact with the magnet is slowly shifted up the side of the tube to the top. The influence of iron particles is serious enough that some careful workers prefer to handle materials for NMR samples with spatulas made of silver rather than of nickel or stainless steel.

Filtration of the Sample Solution

Since solids give extremely broad lines in the NMR spectrum, the presence of small amounts of suspended solid material in the sample does not normally affect the appearance of the average spectrum. However, since solid impurities may be ferromagnetic, it is recommended that sample solutions for NMR spectroscopy routinely be filtered. Figure 8-3a illustrates a small filtering device which can be used to filter the solution as it is added to the sample tube.

Another convenient method is to put a small glass wool plug in the narrow portion of a medicine dropper (Figure 8-3b). The glass wool acts as a filter with small solvent hold up. The dropper and plug can also serve as a weighing boat. Small filters are available which fit the hub of a syringe. The sample solution may be drawn into the the syringe, the filter attached, and the solution expressed through the filter into the NMR sample tube. Another procedure is to make up

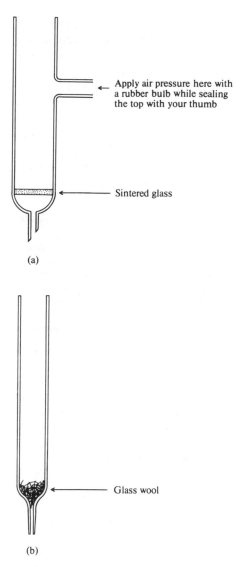

Figure 8-3   Filters for Sample Solutions.

the solution in a small centrifuge cone, centrifuge it, and then transfer the liquid to the NMR tube with a dropper. With finely divided impurities, centrifugation is much faster than filtration.

8.2   SAMPLE TUBE

The basic requirements for the sample container used in NMR spectrometry are that it (1) fit in the receiver coil and (2) be nonmetallic. A long glass tube sealed at one end satisfies these requirements. However, to improve resolution by averaging out some of the residual non-homogeneity of the applied magnetic field, the sample is spun at 20 to 60 Hz, and the tube must therefore be able to be spun smoothly about its long axis so that the receiver coil will not be damaged. In addition, the tube must be symmetrical in cross section, both internally and externally, in order to maximize resolution and minimize spinning sidebands (see Section 9.1). For maximum sensitivity, especially with dilute solutions, as high a "filling factor" as possible is desired, i.e., as much sample is to be concentrated in the active volume of the receiver coil as possible and the air space and container volume are to be kept at a minimum. To meet all these requirements, a precision, thin-walled glass tube is used; typical specifications for the common 5 mm NMR tube are given in Table 8-1.

Table 8-1   Typical Specifications for the 5 mm NMR Sample Tube

Tube length	7.25″		
Outside diameter	0.196″	+0.000	−0.001
Inside diameter	0.161″	+0.000	−0.001

Outside diameter variation over the length of the tube: less than 0.0005″

Camber (or "bow" or "arching") over the length of the tube: less than 0.003″

The more common NMR spectrometers available to the organic chemist are limited to the 5 mm sample tube. However, many of the research spectrometers are able to accommodate larger diameter sample tubes, up to 15 mm in some cases. In situations where only dilute solutions can be obtained, the larger diameter sample tube significantly increases the sensitivity; the increase is roughly in proportion to the square of the radius.

Vortex Plugs

When the sample tube is spun in the probe, a vortex or whirlpool will develop at the top of the solution and can lead to loss of resolution (section 9.1). With large diameter tubes or with small sample volumes the problem can be especially severe. To minimize the problem, a "vortex plug" can be slipped into the tube with the help of a threaded, removable rod. Placing the plug against the top of the solution prevents the vortex from forming.

Special Tubes

A number of types of special NMR tubes are available. With a fused quartz tube, a photochemical reaction can be carried out in the tube and the progress of the reaction followed by NMR without having to transfer the solution. Conversely, an amberized tube can be used with photosensitive samples.

For samples which react with glass, a plastic insert can be used.

For semimicro work, several types of tubes are availabe. One is similar to an ordinary NMR tube but has thick walls and a capillary bore. The sample is gotten to the bottom of the tube by shaking it down as with a fever thermometer. Another has a narrow capillary tube attached to the bottom of a larger tube that slides inside a normal NMR tube. The capillary section can contain a standard solution, a small quantity of a neat liquid, or a small quantity of a concentrated solution. All small capacity tubes are hard to clean.

Sample Tube Stoppers

Sample tubes are always closed in some way before being placed in the instrument. The commercially available plastic caps or serum stoppers are quite convenient and, unlike cork stoppers, they do not shred. Different colored caps can be used to distinguish samples. Neither plastic caps nor rubber stoppers are impervious to solvent vapors, and solvent will gradually evaporate during storage. Sample tubes are thin walled and fragile; caps must be put on and removed with care.

Mixing the Solution

Since NMR tubes are long and narrow, it is difficult to mix the sample and solvent in the tube. To ensure thorough mixing, especially with a relatively viscous solvent such as dimethylsulfoxide, the tube should be inverted several times and the contents allowed to run from one end to the other. An incompletely mixed sample will give a poorly resolved spectrum.

Cleaning Sample Tubes

Since NMR tubes are expensive ($2 to $5), they are cleaned and reused whenever possible. The best way to clean the tube is to rinse it with solvent immediately after use. Chromic acid cleaning solutions should never be used since it is easy to leave behind a trace of paramagnetic chromium ions that will result in line-broadening with subsequent samples.

There are a number of tube cleaning devices available. They help by speeding up the cleaning and rinsing processes.

Labeling the Tube

If a tube is labeled, the label should go all the way around but not overlap. Otherwise the tube may not spin smoothly, resulting in strong spinning sidebands (see Section 9.1) or, in an extreme case, in breaking of the tube. It is best not to use labels but to distinguish samples by using caps of different colors.

8.3 SOLVENTS

As explained in Section 8.1, the substance to be studied by high resolution NMR spectroscopy must be sampled as a liquid or as a solution. Even liquids must be used in solution if reliable chemical shift data are desired.

The ideal solvent for NMR spectroscopy will not contain the nucleus being studied in the sample (so that the solvent will not absorb in the region of interest); it will have a low viscosity (so that intermolecular interactions will be averaged out by random molecular motion), and it will be a good solublizer (because relatively high concentrations are needed—50 mg./0.5 ml. corresponds to 10 grams/100 ml). For proton NMR spectroscopy, carbon tetrachloride (CCl_4) and carbon disulfide (CS_2) fulfill the requirements of no protons in the solvent and of low viscosity, but they are not good solvents for the more polar organic substances often encountered. Chloroform ($CHCl_3$) is a good solvent for a wide variety of organic compounds and is nonviscous, but it contains a proton. It is possible to obtain deuterochloroform ($CDCl_3$) in bulk for about 10¢ per gram, and this substance, which has all the virtues required of a proton NMR solvent, is the most widely used.

If the substance is so slightly soluble in the preferred solvents, $CDCl_3$, CCl_4, and CS_2, that the concentration is below that which can be satisfactorily detected by the NMR spectrometer, there are several courses of action. The easiest is to try additional solvents such as acetone, acetonitrile, pyridine, dimethyl sulfoxide, formamide, or trifluoroacetic acid, as well as water and methanol. All of these can be obtained with deuterium in place of hydrogen, although at a higher price. Some of the properties of these solvents are given later in Table 8-2. The preliminary solubility tests can, of course, be made using non-deuterated solvents, but the deuterated analog is usually to be preferred for obtaining the spectrum, despite the expense. The primary asset of deuterated solvents is that no portion of the spectrum is obscured either by the absorption bands of the solvent or by the spinning sidebands of the extremely strong solvent peak. Furthermore, integration using a nondeuterated solvent is more difficult since the phase detector of the spectrometer must be set extremely accurately; if this is not done, a small amount of the "dispersion mode" from the intense solvent peak will appear as "drift" a considerable distance from the band center (see Section 9.3). Of course, if a high quality spectrum is not required, or if the solvents cannot readily be obtained in deuterated form, spectra of the compound in two or more solvents may be obtained and pieced together.

A second possible solution to the problem of a slightly soluble substance is to dissolve the sample in the NMR tube at a high temperature and then cool the sample and obtain the spectrum of the supersaturated solution. If care is taken to eliminate small crystals which serve as seeds, the solution will remain considerably supersaturated for a surprisingly long time.

The most commonly used deuterated solvent is deuterochloroform; it is relatively inexpensive and is a good solvent for many types of organic compounds. It usually contains a small amount of ordinary chloroform ($CHCl_3$) and, if so, its resonance may be seen at high spectrometer amplitudes at $\delta = 7.27$. Since chloroform is unstable in the presence of moisture and oxygen, it is a wise precaution, for the most careful work, to purify the chloroform immediately before use by passing it through a short column of neutral alumina in a small chromatographic column made from a medicine dropper and a bit of glass wool. This procedure will also remove the ethanol that is sometimes added to normal chloroform as a stabilizer. If the ethanol is not removed, it will be seen at high spectrometer amplitudes.

Hexadeuteroacetone $\left(\begin{matrix} & O \\ & \parallel \\ CD_3 & -C-CD_3 \end{matrix} \right)$ is a good solvent for many substances, as is trideuteroacetonitrile ($CD_3C \equiv N$). Hexadeuterodimethylsulfoxide $\left(\begin{matrix} & O \\ & \parallel \\ CD_3 & -S-CD_3 \end{matrix} \right)$ is a good solvent for many polar substances, but has the disadvantages of being hygroscopic and somewhat viscous. The higher viscosity results in slightly broadened spectral peaks and poorer resolution. In all three of these solvents, the residual protons are, on the average, coupled to two deuterium atoms with $J = 1$ to 2 Hz and will appear as a closely spaced $1:2:3:2:1$ quintet.

Deuterated trifluoroacetic acid $\left(\begin{matrix} & O \\ & \parallel \\ CF_3 & -C-OD \end{matrix} \right)$ is an excellent solvent for basic compounds since it is a strong acid. Because of protonation of the molecule, nuclei at or near the site of protonation may be strongly deshielded.

Both deuterium oxide (D_2O) and deuteriomethanol (CD_3OD) are excellent solvents for highly polar substances. If poor results are obtained with deuterium oxide, distillation of the solvent may improve matters considerably. Samples of heavy water have been obtained in which suspended ferric oxide was visible. A disadvantage of these two solvents, as well as of deuterotrifluoacetic acid, is that they will replace all $-OH$ and $-NH$ protons in the sample molecules with deuterium. Consequently, all such protons will give a common singlet at the chemical shift for the $-OH$ protons of the solvent.

Spectra obtained using an aromatic compound as solvent should be interpreted with caution if only the one solvent is used. Both specific solvation and diamagnetic anisotropy can cause relatively large solvent effects that make comparison of chemical shift data with data obtained with "normal" solvents difficult. Pyridine presents a predicament: it is an excellent solvent for many compounds, but it is also both a weak base and an aromatic system and it produces solvent shifts on the order of 0.2 to 0.3 ppm. If pyridine or other aromatic solvents are used, it is recommended that model compounds (if they are available) also be studied in the same solvents as well as in more normal solvents. In this way, some estimate of the magnitude of the solvent effect will be available.

The water-miscible solvents present a storage problem in that they readily pick up water vapor from the air. They should be stored in tightly closed containers, preferably in a desiccator. A convenient desiccator for this purpose is a small, wide-mouth screw top jar with some indicating Drierite in the bottom.

If necessary, wet solvents can be dried by chromatography on a small amount of activated molecular sieve.

Table 8-2 shows some of the properties of the solvents most commonly used in proton NMR spectroscopy.

Table 8-2 Selected Properties of Some Common Proton NMR Solvents

Compounds	Melting point	Boiling point	Resonance, δ	Cost, $/gram*
Carbon tetrachloride	−23	77	—	—
Chloroform	−64	61	7.27	7/50
Carbon disulfide	−104	46	—	—
Benzene	5	80	7.20	8/5
Acetone	−95	57	2.05	6/5
Acetonitrile	−42	82	1.98	9/5
p-Dioxane	12	101	3.55	20/1
Methanol	−98	65	3.35 (CH_3) ~4.8 (OH; variable)	33/5
Water	0	100	~4.8 (variable)	
Deuterium oxide	+3.8	101.4	~4.8 (variable)	18/100
Dichloromethane	−95	40	5.35	26/5
Pyridine	−42	115	6.9–8.5	17/5
Trifluoroacetic acid	−15	74	12.5 (variable)	8/5
Dimethylsulfoxide	18	189	2.58	6/5
Sulfur dioxide	−72	−10	—	—

* Cost is for the fully deuterated analog.

It is not recommended that samples be stored in solution with the thought of running the spectrum weeks later for comparison. Chloroform, for example, is not stable in the presence of moisture and oxygen; it forms phosgene in such an environment. In addition, it reacts slowly with amines and other compounds, especially in the presence of oxygen. If you want to try to save a sample in chloroform solution, it must be degassed, and the tube must be stored at a low temperature.

8.4   REFERENCE STANDARDS

Since the strength of the magnetic field employed in proton magnetic resonance spectroscopy cannot be measured with the required accuracy of about 1 part in 10^8, the peak of an arbitrary reference substance must be used as a point of origin from which line positions may be measured for comparison between compounds and investigators.

A practical secondary use of the reference standard is as a check upon both the instrument and the solution. All the recommended standards possess very narrow intrinsic line widths, and therefore the resolution of the instrument may be quickly noted by the appearance of the reference peak. The position and relative size of the spinning side-bands can also be checked, and since they will be reasonably constant over the entire spectrum, they can easily be identified.

Tetramethylsilane (TMS) is a volatile (b.p. = 26°C.), symmetrical, inert substance that is miscible with most organic solvents, thus fulfilling the require-

$$
\begin{array}{c}
CH_3 \\
| \\
CH_3 - Si - CH_3 \\
| \\
CH_3
\end{array}
$$

tetramethylsilane (TMS)

ments of a proton standard quite admirably. In addition, its resonance is a very sharp singlet somewhat removed to higher field from the resonances of most other organic protons. Therefore the proposal that this substance be used as the primary internal standard for proton resonance spectroscopy has gained wide acceptance.

The simplest way to establish a reference is to add a small amount of the reference substance to the NMR tube containing the sample solution. A satisfactory concentration of TMS is usually between 1 and 3 percent, or 0.005 to 0.015 ml/0.5 ml of solvent. A 0.10 ml syringe is useful for accurately adding TMS or another standard to the NMR tube. We have found that keeping the TMS in a stoppered serum vial and storing the vial and the syringe in the refrigerator makes the transfer of the volatile TMS to the sample tube a very simple operation. However, many of the suppliers of deuterated solvents will supply the solvent with TMS present, or TMS can be added locally.

As secondary standards, cyclohexane or hexamethyldisiloxane are employed.

$$
\begin{array}{cc}
CH_3 & CH_3 \\
| & | \\
CH_3 \ Si \ \ O - Si - CH_3 \\
| & | \\
CH_3 & CH_3
\end{array}
$$

hexamethyldisiloxane

They are easier to handle than TMS at room temperature (especially during the summer) and both are of use at higher temperatures where TMS tends to "boil out" of solution. TMS is preferred for use in acidic solutions due to the possibility of the oxygen of hexamethyldisiloxane associating with proton donors, but even TMS cannot be used in concentrated sulfuric acid.

The preceding standards are all insoluble in water, and therefore other compounds must be used in this medium. As the primary standard for aqueous solution, sodium trimethylsilylpropane sulfonate is gaining acceptance. This

$$
\begin{array}{c}
CH_3 \\
| \\
CH_3 - Si - CH_2CH_2CH_2 - SO_3^- Na^+ \\
| \\
CH_3
\end{array}
$$

sodium trimethylsilylpropane sulfonate

compound is also available with the protons on the methylene groups replaced by deuterium. Dioxane and acetonitrile have also been suggested.

If sample absorption is anticipated in the region of reference absorption, the spectrum should first be studied without the standard present. When the region of reference absorption has been checked for peaks, the standard can be added with the assurance that it is not obscuring any sample peaks.

If deuterochloroform is the solvent, the normal chloroform impurity which shows up at about $\delta = 7.27$ can be used as a rough internal standard.

If the standards mentioned above are inadequate, the reference material selected for use as an internal standard should not be capable of associating with either the solvent or the compounds being studied. If in doubt, two or more standards can be used; a variation of chemical shift differences between reference peaks will indicate that at least one reference is subject to association.

Water is sometimes used as a standard, especially in D_2O, but the position of the water resonance is very sensitive to both temperature and pH.

Table 8-3 gives the position of the resonance of several possible reference compounds relative to TMS as 0.00.

Table 8-3 Chemical Shifts of Reference Compounds for Proton NMR Relative to TMS

Compound	δ
Tetramethylsilane	0.00
Sodium trimethylsilylpropane sulfonate	0.00 ± 0.02
Hexamethyldisiloxane	0.06
Silicone stopcock grease	0.1
Cyclohexane	1.44
Chloroform	7.27 (slightly variable)
Acetonitrile	1.98
Dioxane	3.7
Water	4.8 (variable)
Tetramethylammonium bromide	3.10

9 Operation of the NMR Spectrometer

In this chapter we will consider some of the practical aspects of the operation of the NMR spectrometer. Section 9.1 will describe the instrument settings generally required for obtaining a routine proton NMR spectrum. The remaining sections will consider some of the less routine, more demanding procedures such as determination and optimization of the magnetic field homogeneity and resolving power of the instrument, integration of the spectra, and calibration of the spectrum.

9.1 SETTING UP THE NMR SPECTROMETER FOR A ROUTINE SPECTRUM

Since each instrument has its own operating characteristics, we can give only some general suggestions concerning the various adjustments or settings that must be made. After describing the various operating parameters, we will briefly outline how to obtain a routine spectrum.

Sweep Width

For the first proton NMR spectrum of an unknown compound, a sweep width of about 10 ppm from $\delta = 10$ to 0 ($\tau = 0$ to 10) is appropriate. This will correspond to a sweep width of 600 Hz with a 60 MHz instrument (see Figure 3-3). With subsequent spectra, a smaller sweep width may be used in order to better observe parts of the spectrum. Since the scan will always run from one end of the chart paper to the other, use of a smaller sweep width amounts to stretching the spectrum along the chemical shift axis.

Sweep Offset

If you think of the sweep width as a "window" through which you look at the spectrum, the sweep offset is the adjustment used to move this window along the chemical shift axis so that you can see that portion of the spectrum that interests you. For the first proton NMR spectrum of an unknown compound, the 10 ppm portion of greatest interest is from $\delta = 10$ to 0 ($\tau = 0$ to 10); a sweep offset setting of zero will place the 10 ppm window over this portion of the spectrum.

Whenever the sweep offset is set at zero, 0 of the δ scale and 10 of the τ scale will be at the right hand side of the scan for all sweep widths (i.e., no matter what size the window is, the TMS resonance will always lie at the right-hand side when the sweep offset is set at zero). Therefore to look at a portion of the spectrum beyond the left hand side of the window, the sweep offset must be turned to slide the spectrum to the right. For example, if with a sweep width of 10 ppm you wish to look at the portion of the spectrum from $\delta = 15$ to 5 ($\tau = -5$ to $+5$), a sweep offset of $+5$ ppm would be needed; this would correspond to a setting of 150 Hz for a 30 MHz instrument or 300 Hz for a 60 MHz instrument.

Sweep Zero

As we have just said, for all sweep widths, when the sweep offset is set at zero, the TMS resonance will lie at the right side or at the zero of precalibrated chart paper. If it does not fall exactly at the zero, the sweep zero is used to slide the spectrum along the chemical shift axis until the TMS resonance does lie exactly at the zero. If a different reference standard is employed, the sweep zero is used to place its resonance at the proper position on the chemical shift axis. Table 8-3 gives the position of resonance of some other standards relative to TMS as 0.00.

Sweep Time

The setting of the sweep time determines the rate at which the portion of the spectrum in the window is scanned. The rate of scan equals the sweep width divided by the sweep time (Hz/sec). A typical rate of scan is about 1 Hz/sec. If the total sweep width is 600 Hz (10 ppm in a 60 MHz instrument), an appropriate sweep time would be 600 seconds (10 minutes).

Too rapid scanning will cause the peaks to appear distorted because of the inability of the recorder pen to respond rapidly enough.

Too slow scanning can lead to saturation (see Section 2.3) since the longer the time of irradiation of the magnetically active nuclei, the greater will be the rf energy input. At higher rf fields, the rate of scan must be greater to avoid saturation (the scan time must be smaller).

rf Power

Up to a point, increasing the rf (radio frequency) power will give a stronger spectrum since it is the source of the energy which causes the transitions between nuclear spin states. Eventually, however, saturation will set in (see Section 2.3) and further increases in the rf power will lead to a shortened and broadened peak. Figure 9-1 shows the variation in appearance of the resonance of $CHCl_3$ as the rf power is increased while all other operating parameters are held constant. The point at which a further increase in rf power will lead to a loss of peak height rather than a gain can be determined only by repeated scans at increasing rf power.

It is important to remember that saturation will occur at a different rf power for nuclei at different chemical shifts, even in the same molecule. In general, nuclei that give sharp, narrow peaks tend to saturate more easily. It is also observed that at lower rates of scan, saturation occurs at lower rf powers since the lower rate of scan exposes the nuclei to more rf radiation. Thus there will be an optimum rf power for maximum sensitivity that will depend both upon the particular magnetically active nuclei involved and upon the rate of scan.

Spectrum Amplitude

The spectrum amplitude is usually set so that the strongest peak in the spectrum spans the full height of the chart. The required setting is determined by trial and error.

Filter

The filter refers to an electronic circuit used to remove some of the high frequency noise present in the detector circuits. It becomes desirable to do this

Figure 9-1 Appearance of the Resonance of $CHCl_3$ as a Function of Increasing rf Power.

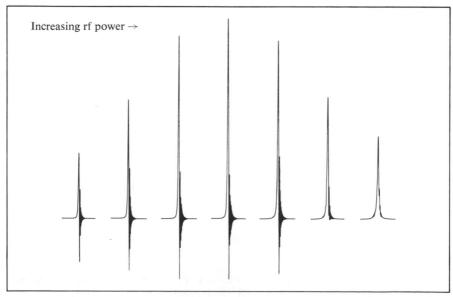

Increasing rf power →

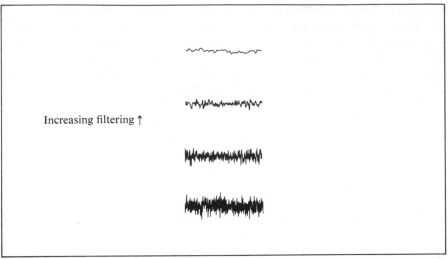

Figure 9-2   Effect of Increased Filtering on Baseline Noise.

when operating at higher spectrum amplitudes. Figure 9-2 shows the smoothing effect that increased filtering has on the baseline noise. Figure 9-3 shows the change in the appearance of the sharp $CHCl_3$ resonance that accompanies increased filtering.

In addition to smoothing out noise, some filtering may be desirable in order to partially damp out ringing.* If peaks are closely spaced, the ringing from one may partially overlap the next. However, since filtering dampens the motion of

Figure 9-3   Appearance of the Resonance of $CHCl_3$ as a Function of Increased Filtering.

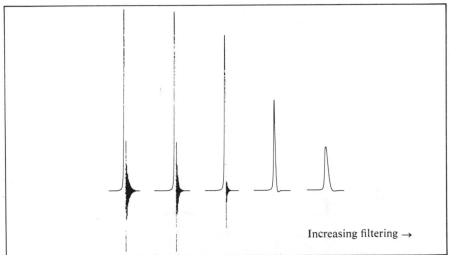

* "Ringing" is a smoothly decaying pen oscillation that appears after passage through a sharp resonance peak when the magnetic field homogeneity is high.

the pen, the peaks soon become distorted, as can be seen in Figure 9-3, and therefore lower rates of scan must be used with increased filtering. With the lower rate of scan, the rf power may also have to be reduced to avoid saturation. The setting of the filter (in seconds) should be no greater than the rate of scan (in Hz/second). Thus for the usual rate of scan of about 1 Hz/sec, the filter should be set to a value no greater than 1 sec.

Phase (Signal Symmetry)

The symmetry of the absorption peak is determined by the phase adjustment. Figure 9-4 shows the appearance of the resonance of the $CHCl_3$ peak as a function of the phase setting. A slight change in the phase setting may be needed when the rf power, spectrum amplitude, or solvent is changed. The phase setting is not especially important when recording the absorption spectrum, but it is critical when recording the integral.

Spinning the Sample

In order to partially average out residual magnetic field nonhomogeneity, the tube containing the sample is spun about its long axis. This is accomplished by fitting the tube with a plastic turbine that is powered by compressed air in the probe. The position of the turbine is set with a depth gauge, and the spin rate is determined by the rate of flow of the compressed air. Figure 9-5 shows the appearance of the resonance of $CHCl_3$ as a function of spinning rate. The extra peaks appearing to each side of the $CHCl_3$ resonance are artifacts resulting from the spinning of the sample; they are called *spinning sidebands*. For a given

Figure 9-4 Appearance of the Resonance of $CHCl_3$ as a Function of Phase Adjustment.

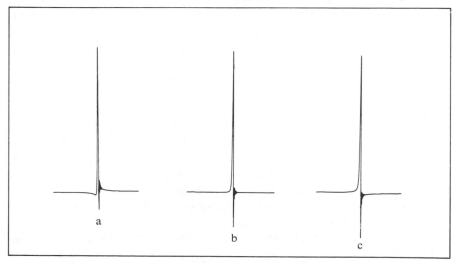

a: clockwise correction needed; b: satisfactory; c: counterclockwise correction needed.

spinning rate, the spinning sidebands are stronger the less homogeneous the magnetic field; if the magnetic field were perfectly homogeneous, there would be no spinning sidebands. The sample may experience a nonhomogeneous magnetic field not only because of nonhomogeneity of the magnetic field but also because of nonuniformity in the wall thickness of the sample tube. For this reason, some tubes will give smaller spinning sidebands than others. A tube which wobbles while spinning will also give larger spinning sidebands. As you can also see from Figure 9-5, the greater the spinning rate, the smaller the spinning sidebands. A spinning rate between 30 and 60 Hz will usually be appropriate. Too great a rate of spinning will cause the depression from the vortex or miniature whirlpool in the solution in the sample tube to dip down into the sensitive volume of the receiver coil; a sudden loss of resolution and sensitivity will result.

If the spinning rate of the sample is known, spinning sidebands are easily identified in a spectrum because they appear spaced out to each side of each peak at a distance equal to or an integral multiple of the spinning rate (as can be seen in Figure 9-5). If you are running the spectrum, you can verify the identity of spinning sidebands by rescanning with a different spinning rate; the spinning sidebands will move to a new position. You must be careful not to confuse spinning sidebands of strong peaks with weak peaks.

In some of the spectra presented as examples in this book, spinning sidebands cannot be seen. This is because we tried to avoid some confusion by scanning over them at a reduced spectrum amplitude.

Fine Y (Resolution; Homogeneity)

Spinning the sample cannot average out magnetic field gradients along the axis of spin (the Y axis). Therefore to optimize the magnetic field homogeneity in this direction, and thereby optimize resolution, slight adjustments can be made to the field along this axis by the Fine Y control. The resolution of the instrument is most sensitive to this control. Figure 9-6 shows the appearance of the resonance of $CHCl_3$ as a function of this adjustment.

Maximum magnetic field homogeneity and therefore resolution is indicated by maximum peak height (and therefore minimum peak width) and by strong ringing. Figure 9-6d shows the $CHCl_3$ resonance when the Fine Y (Resolution) control was set for maximum peak height and best quality of ringing.

The improvement in resolution can be followed by looking either at the increase in peak height or the improvement of the quality of the ringing. Near the optimum setting, only very slight adjustments are needed.

After optimizing resolution by adjusting Fine Y, changing samples (or even removing and immediately replacing the same sample tube) will necessitate retrimming Fine Y for maximum resolution.

In order to attain the best resolution, the sample must be in thermal equilibrium with the probe that supports the sample tube in the instrument. It therefore is a good idea to make the Fine Y (Resolution) adjustment last.

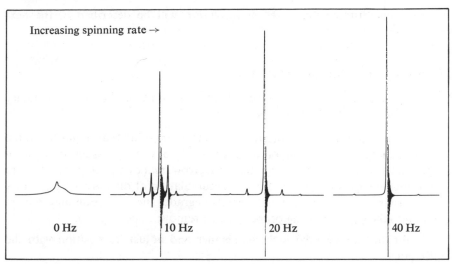

Figure 9-5   Appearance of the Resonance of $CHCl_3$ as a Function of Increasing Spinning Rate.

Figure 9-6   Appearance of the Resonance of $CHCl_3$ as a Function of the Adjustment of Fine Y (Resolution; Homogeneity).

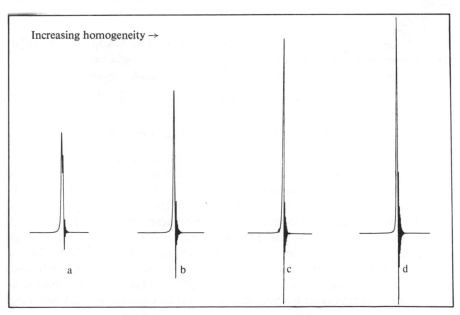

Some quantitative measures of resolution will be described in the next section.

Obtaining a Routine Spectrum

After you have prepared the sample (Chapter 8), you can obtain a preliminary spectrum by using the following procedure:

1. Wipe the sample tube carefully to remove anything that might be on the outside, like spilled solution or fingerprints. Use wiping tissues or a clean handkerchief; if your shirt is clean, the inside front makes a good wiper. Failure to thoroughly wipe the tube leads to an accumulation of dirt, grease, and other residue inside the probe where it ultimately degrades the resolution and impairs spinning to the point that the probe must be removed and cleaned.

2. Fit the sample tube with the spinner and adjust its position with the depth gauge.

3. Rewipe the tube to remove any dust picked up from the depth gauge.

4. Carefully insert the sample tube into the probe assembly and adjust the flow of compressed air to spin the sample tube at 30 to 60 Hz.

5. Set the Sweep Width, the Sweep Offset, and the Sweep Time to the desired values. For an unknown compound, values of 10 ppm or 500 Hz for Sweep Width, zero for Sweep Offset, and 10 minutes or 500 seconds for Sweep Time are appropriate.

6. Set the rf power to the middle of the range (or another recommended value).

7. Set the Filter to its lowest value.

8. If the instrument has a flat bed recorder rather than a strip chart recorder, place a piece of blank paper on the recorder platen or use a printed chart and overlay it with a piece of cheap, translucent paper such as onionskin.

9. Set the Spectrum Amplitude control somewhere in the middle of its range.

10. Activate the spectrometer and scan through the spectrum.

Assuming that you obtain some kind of a spectrum, it is now time to improve it by alternately making various adjustments and rescanning portions of the spectrum until you are satisfied with the results. First, the Spectrum Amplitude will almost certainly need to be adjusted to obtain the desired peak heights. Second, resolution can be optimized by alternately scanning a strong, sharp peak (usually the reference peak) and adjusting Fine Y. Phase can be adjusted although this is usually not necessary, unless you are changing solvents or are making a large change in rf field. Finally, set the resonance of the reference substance to the correct value by means of the Sweep Zero. The reference peak can be identified (1) because it will be near its expected value and (2) because it will be a very sharp peak. This setting is made last since the zero will drift while the sample is coming to thermal equilibrium with the probe. (If the reference is off scale due to the setting of Sweep Offset, set Sweep Offset to zero, set the reference peak with Sweep Zero, and then reset Sweep Offset). Now record the spectrum on the chart. When scanning the reference peak, it may be necessary to momentarily increase the Spectrum Amplitude in order to see the reference peak or to momentarily decrease the Spectrum Amplitude in order to keep it from going off scale.

If you have a dilute sample, it is more difficult to obtain a good spectrum. The rf Power, Spectrum Amplitude, and Filter will all need to be increased; an optimum combination of these settings must be found by trial and error. Saturation must be avoided, as must peak distortion from too much filtering.

For an unknown substance, always check the region between $\delta = 20$ to 10 ($\tau = -10$ to 0). Signals do not often appear in this region, but if you overlook them you will be missing important information.

If you do not obtain a rough spectrum, recheck the instrument settings to be sure that they are what you think they are, and make sure that the sample is spinning. If this does not help, remove your sample and put in a standard sample such as 12 percent TMS in chloroform (sharp singlets at $\delta = 0.00$ and 7.27). By scanning the standard sample, you can assure yourself that the instrument is set up correctly. If you cannot get a spectrum with the standard sample, you need to talk to someone who is familiar with the instrument. If the standard works, then your sample is either too dilute or you may have one of the problems described in Section 8-1. When you fail to obtain a spectrum, the problem is almost always with the sample.

9.2 OPTIMIZING AND MEASURING RESOLUTION

In practical terms, resolution or resolving power is the ability of the spectrometer to distinguish closely spaced peaks. When the intrinsic line width of a peak is small, a measure of the resolving power of a spectrometer is the width of the peak at half height; a minimum value is desired. Figure 9-7 illustrates this measure of resolution. Since improving the resolution makes the absorption peaks taller as well as narrower, it also improves the S/N ratio.

The commonly used internal standard, tetramethylsilane, possesses an intrinsic line width estimated to be 0.02 Hz, but a spectrometer which shows a resolution of 0.1 Hz with this standard is indeed a superior instrument. Resolutions of 0.4 to 0.6 Hz are the norm, and for routine work this is adequate. Except for detailed analysis of spin-spin splitting patterns, splittings of less than about 1.0 Hz are often ignored.

Since tetramethylsilane has such a narrow resonance, it can be used as a quick check of the instrument's condition. A broad TMS signal indicates that something is amiss. When the observed line width of the TMS peak (degassed in an inert solvent) is less than 0.5 Hz, the line width criterion becomes both inaccurate and inconvenient. Optimum resolution can then most conveniently be estimated from the peak height and from the quality of ringing.

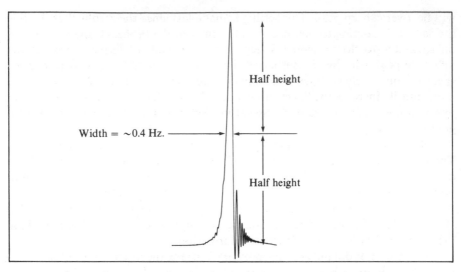

Figure 9-7   Estimation of Resolving Power From Width at Half Height.

Since for precise work, a numerical value for resolution is required, several other tests have gained favor as more exacting checks of the performance of the spectrometer. One standard for resolution is the resonance of the aldehyde proton of neat acetaldehyde $\left(\begin{array}{c} O \\ \parallel \\ CH_3-C-H \end{array}\right)$. This resonance appears at $\delta = 9.80$ as a 1:3:3:1 quartet with a spacing of 2.85 Hz between peaks. Since for this test of resolution the quartet is scanned with a Scan Width of 25 Hz, the Sweep Offset must be set at $+575$ Hz in a 60 MHz instrument. Figure 9-8 shows such a scan of the acetaldehyde quartet. The quality of the resolution is indicated both by the peak width at half height (about 0.3 Hz) and by the good ringing (slow decay and amplitude such that the first upward swing after each of the two middle peaks approximates the height of the two outer peaks).

Resolution must be optimized by alternating small adjustments of Fine Y and scans of the test sample. Near the setting for optimum resolution, the required adjustments are very small indeed, and it is sometimes helpful to wait a few seconds after making the adjustment before running the test scan. If the desired resolution cannot be obtained by adjustment of Fine Y, the instrument should be "tuned" by someone who is thoroughly familiar with its characteristics. Remember, almost all difficulties in obtaining a spectrum are due to the sample and not the instrument.

Tuning for maximum resolution takes time, but fortunately maximum resolving power is not often needed. A relatively quick and satisfactory method for tuning the Varian T-60 is to:

1. Scan the acetaldehyde quartet with the following instrumental settings:

Filter: 1
Spectrum Amplitude: 5.0
rf Power: 0.01
Sweep Time: 250 seconds
Sweep Width: 25 Hz
Sweep Offset: 575 Hz (approximately, depending upon how accurately
                             TMS has been set on zero)

2. Set the rf Power to 0.0075, the Spectrum Amplitude to 1, disable the field sweep by releasing all Sweep Widths buttons, and switch from Operate to Adjust.

3. Then while scanning with the 250 second Sweep Time, *slowly* adjust Resolution (Fine Y) to give maximum upward pen deflection. In a rare instance, a minute change in Curvature is helpful.

4. Switch from Adjust to Operate, reset to the conditions of (1), and rescan the acetaldehyde quartet.

It is important to remember that to achieve the best possible resolution, the sample must be in thermal equilibrium with the probe.

Even after obtaining the desired resolution, as indicated by any of the tests mentioned, the magnetic field must be retrimmed after the sample is placed in the probe if maximum resolution is desired (because of differences in magnetic properties between different solvents and different sample tubes).

Figure 9-8   Estimation of the Resolving Power of an NMR Spectrometer from the Aldehyde Quartet of Acetaldehyde.

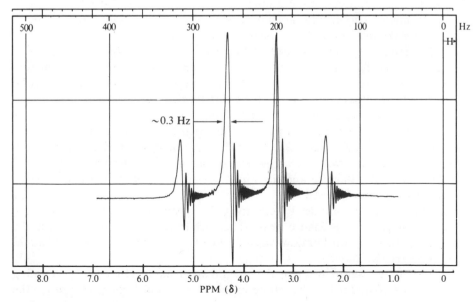

9.3 INTEGRATION OF THE SPECTRUM

Compared to obtaining the absorption spectrum, integration of the spectrum to obtain relative peak areas is somewhat more demanding, and careful work is required to obtain meaningful data.

While dilute solutions are recommended in order to obtain the most reliable chemical shift data, as concentrated a sample as can be obtained is recommended for integration. With more dilute samples, the larger rf powers required lead to saturation, and with the higher spectrum amplitudes, erratic drifts and noise become more noticeable. In addition, impurities in the solvent, such as the residual protium compounds in deuterated solvents, are less troublesome with concentrated solution. With dilute solutions, a sample that will not yield a satisfactory integral can give an adequate absorption spectrum.

A high rf power is desirable in order to obtain the most favorable S/N ratio. However, saturation must be avoided since it leads to errors in peak area ratios. The optimum rf power is determined by making repeated scans of the portions of the spectrum of interest at higher and higher rf powers. Eventually a point will be reached where peak heights will not increase with the increase in rf power. Saturation has become significant at this point, and the rf power should be backed off somewhat. For best results, each resonance of interest must be checked for saturation since some nuclei saturate more easily than others. Since the presence of dissolved oxygen in the sample tends to shorten and equalize relaxation times (reduce and equalize tendencies toward saturation), degassing of samples for integration is not recommended.

After optimizing the rf power, a rough integral is obtained by scanning in the Integrate mode. The integral must be scanned rapidly in order to minimize pen drift and, more importantly, random changes in pen drift; a sweep time of 1/5 to 1/10 of that used for the scanning of the absorption spectrum will usually be appropriate. The integral amplitude is adjusted for additional trial scans in order to make maximum use of the chart height.

The remaining problems are to adjust the Phase and Balance (Drift and Zero) controls. The Phase control is the same one which was discussed in Section 9-1. When these controls are both set correctly, the integral trace will be perfectly horizontal before and after the vertical rise for each peak (see Figure 9-9b). If the Balance is not set correctly, there will be an upward or downward drift to all the horizontal parts of the spectrum although they will still be parallel (see Figure 9-9c and 9-9d). If the Phase is not set correctly, the horizontal parts of the integral will not be parallel to one another (see Figures 9-10 and 9-11). If both the Balance and the Phase are set incorrectly, the two types of errors will be superimposed.

The Balance is best set by offsetting the spectrum so that the pen is far removed from any resonance peak. Then while scanning slowly, adjust the Balance until no upward or downward drift can be detected. The Balance should be set before the Phase.

The Phase is set by scanning the integral and making adjustments according to Figures 9-10 and 9-11. The setting of the Phase is much more critical for the

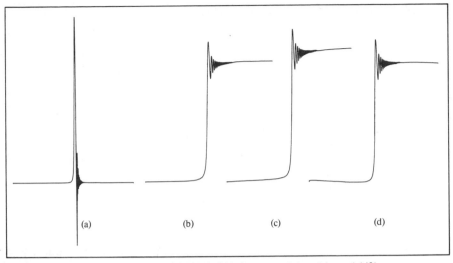

(a) Absorption spectrum   (c) Integral of (a): detector not balanced (upward drift)
(b) Integral of (a): detector balanced   (d) Integral of (a): detector not balanced (downward drift)

Figure 9-9   Optimum Detector Phase Setting.

appearance of the integral than for the absorption spectrum; as you can see from Figures 9-10 and 9-11, the maladjustment of the Phase is scarcely noticeable in the absorption spectrum but is very obvious in the integral.

Figure 9-10   Incorrect Detector Phase Setting.

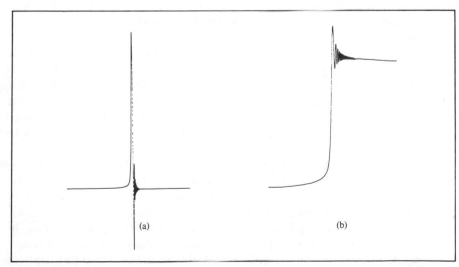

(a) Absorption spectrum
(b) Integral of (a): counterclockwise phase correction needed

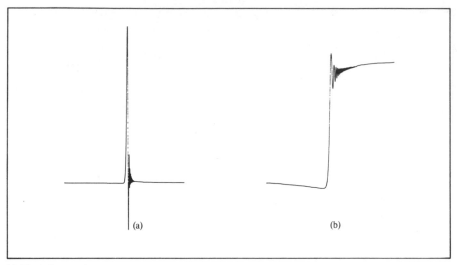

(a) Absorption spectrum
(b) Integral of (a): clockwise phase correction needed

Figure 9-11   Incorrect Detector Phase Setting.

If it is impossible to make the integral trace horizontal both before and after the vertical rise by adjustment of Phase, the Balance is not set properly. Since a maladjustment of Phase shows up as drift a considerable distance from the peak, Balance must be set when the pen is offset as far as possible from any resonance peak. If the rf power or the spectrum amplitude is changed, Balance and Phase will have to be reset.

After the instrument has been set up, the integral should be recorded several times in both directions in order to average the results. A pause of about a minute between passes is recommended to allow relaxation and avoid saturation.

The height of the vertical rise in the integral trace is proportional to the number of magnetically active nuclei responsible for the resonance. For each set of magnetically active nuclei, all the peaks of the multiplet must be included, as well as the spinning sidebands. Since the estimate of the relative areas of the resonances depends upon the accuracy with which the vertical rises can be measured, it is a good idea to use a higher integral amplitude and to reset the trace to the baseline between resonances, whenever possible.

A nonspinning sample can yield a more accurate integral than a spinning sample. If the peaks are widely spaced, optimum resolution is not needed and the instrument may be adjusted for best nonspinning resolution. Usually three to four Hz nonspinning resolution can be obtained, and it is possible to obtain better values with some magnets. If the peaks are closely spaced, it may be necessary to spin the sample to obtain the required resolution. If the field homogeneity is high, ringing can be seen in both the absorption spectrum and the integral (Figures 9-9 through 9-11).

When you need to integrate closely spaced peaks, it will be helpful to adjust the Fine Y to slightly degrade the resolution and thus to eliminate most of the ringing. This will make it easier to measure the step heights of the integral trace.

If maximum sensitivity is required, you can take advantage of the fact that the integral is scanned faster than the absorption spectrum and increase the rf power by the square root of the increase in the rate of scan. For example, if the scan time for the integration is one-tenth that at which the optimum rf power setting was determined for the absorption spectrum, the rf power may be increased by a factor of $\sqrt{10}$ (or about 3) when the integral is scanned.

The absence of saturation effects can be confirmed by redetermining the integral as a slightly lower setting of the rf power and seeing that the relative peak areas are unchanged. If they do change, further determinations at still lower rf powers must be made. Each change of rf power may necessitate adjustment of both Balance and Phase for best results.

9.4 CALIBRATION OF THE SPECTRUM

Calibration is the procedure by which you ensure that the estimates of peak positions on the chemical shift axis of the absorption spectrum are sufficiently accurate for the purpose for which the spectrum is being determined.

For routine comparison and interpretation of NMR spectra, such as in qualitative organic analysis, an accuracy of ± 1 or 2 Hz from the "true" peak position is entirely adequate. One normally assumes that the spectrometer is operating with at least this accuracy, but this assumption can easily be checked by determining the spectrum of a sample for which peak positions are assumed to be accurately known. For example, the peaks of a solution of 12 percent TMS in chloroform appear at $\delta = 0.00$ and $\delta = 7.27$ (or 436 Hz apart in a 60 MHz instrument).

The accuracy of the calibration of the Sweep Offset can be checked to ± 1 Hz by recording the TMS resonance of the 12 percent TMS in chloroform sample, setting the Sweep Offset to $+436$ Hz (in a 60 MHz instrument) and recording the chloroform resonance. The two peaks should coincide (assuming no drift of the spectrum along the chemical shift axis during the time between recording the two peaks.)

Using this same TMS/chloroform sample, the accuracy of the calibration of the expanded scales can be tested to ± 1 Hz by adjusting the TMS resonance to $\delta = 0.00$ by means of the Sweep Zero control, setting the Sweep Offset to the value theoretically required to place the chloroform resonance at the left hand side of the chart for the expanded sweep width (e.g., Sweep Offset = 186 for Sweep Width = 250 Hz), and recording the chloroform resonance. The chloroform resonance should appear at $+436$ Hz which exactly equals the Sweep Width plus the Sweep Offset (again assuming no drift).

In all procedures just described, drift along the chemical shift axis during the time between recordings of different peaks will show up as an apparent calibration error. Drift can be estimated by recording the same peak with the same instrument settings after two to five minute time intervals. If there is observable drift, checking the calibration of Sweep Width and Sweep Offset by the methods just described is not very reliable. It is possible for an instrument to be calibrated accurately but to drift badly.

The major cause of drift is temperature changes in the magnet. This drift can be minimized by holding the temperature of the room as constant as possible, by making sure that air conditioners or heaters do not blow on the instrument, and by adjusting the temperature of the sample to the temperature of the probe. Some instruments have a place to store samples that is kept at the probe temperature. For spectrometers operating at a probe temperature of 35°C, you can warm or cool the sample tube with your hand; be sure to wipe the tube well before putting it into the instrument.

10 Epilogue

In this short book we have been able only to begin to describe some of the ways in which NMR spectroscopy can yield information about molecular structure. We have made no mention at all of other applications of NMR spectroscopy such as quantitative analysis or kinetics, nor have we described such interesting phenomena as the variation of spectra with temperature and solvent, ^{13}C satellites in proton NMR spectra, NMR spectroscopy of magnetic nuclei other than the proton, or how it is possible to determine enantiomeric purity by NMR. In this chapter we will give a very brief indication of the nature and value of some of these other aspects of NMR spectroscopy.

HIGH-FIELD HIGH-FREQUENCY SPECTROMETERS

When it is important to obtain as much structural information as possible from NMR spectroscopy, the spectrum can be determined using a spectrometer with a very intense magnetic field. Routine NMR spectrometers operate at 60 MHz and 14,092 gauss, but instruments operating at 100 MHz and about 23,000 gauss are fairly common, and there are a few spectrometers that operate at 300 MHz using a superconducting solenoid of about 70,000 gauss. When magnetic equivalence is involved, as explained in Chapter 5, a larger H_{ext} will always increase the $\Delta\delta/J$ ratio and thus simplify the spectrum. If magnetic equivalence is not involved, however, this technique will not necessarily result in a simple spectrum. Since the sensitivity of the NMR method increases with increasing H_{ext}, smaller or more dilute samples can be used with the higher field instruments. The study of biopolymers (such as enzymes) has been greatly facilitated by the availability of high-field spectrometers.

SPIN-DECOUPLING

An important technique for simplifying NMR spectra involves irradiating nuclei at one chemical shift with intense rf radiation at their resonance frequency while simultaneously scanning the resonance of other nuclei at a different chemical shift. This technique serves to "decouple" the scanned nuclei from any splitting due to the irradiated nuclei and thus both simplifies the spectrum and indicates which nuclei are mutually coupled. Such "spin decoupling" can be carried out to eliminate the coupling of protons with protons (an example of homonuclear spin decoupling) or the effect of other magnetically active nuclei such as ^{19}F on protons (heteronuclear spin decoupling).

COMPUTER TECHNIQUES

Computer techniques are also widely used in NMR spectroscopy. Programs have been written which take experimental line positions and intensities as input and produce both a table of chemical shift differences and coupling constants, and a plot of a simulated NMR spectrum calculated on the basis of these values as output. If the plotted spectrum looks like the experimental spectrum, one assumes that the calculated chemical shift differences and coupling constants are those of the unknown substance.

A second type of computer technique involves a completely different method of obtaining the NMR spectrum. Instead of using an extremely narrow band of continuous rf radiation centered at the resonance frequency and slowly increasing H_{ext} in order to bring the differently shielded nuclei into resonance, the magnetic field is held constant, and a brief, very intense, pulse of rf power is applied. The bandwidth of the pulse is sufficiently great that nuclei at all chemical shifts are simultaneously excited. The subsequent relaxation produces a very complex interference pattern (ringing) which is the Fourier transform of the normal "continuous wave" (CW) spectrum. The computer stores the interference patterns from many successive pulses (one every two seconds or so), averages them to reduce noise, and finally calculates and displays the corresponding continuous wave spectrum from the accumulated Fourier transforms. Since all the magnetically active nuclei are excited simultaneously every two seconds, rather than, typically, only once during a 500 second scan, many more spectra can be obtained and averaged in a given length of time. The Fourier transform (FT) technique results in a 20- to 30-fold increase in sensitivity, or gives a corresponding decrease in the length of time needed to obtain a useful spectrum.

QUANTITATIVE ANALYSIS

The integral trace of the proton NMR spectrum of a mixture can provide information as to the relative amounts of the components. In a mixture of A and B, for example, if the step height for the integral of a methyl resonance of compound A is 20 units while the step height for the integral of a methyl resonance of compound B is 10 units, there must be twice as much A as B in the sample. Quantitative analysis by this technique is especially useful when the components of the mixture are difficult or impossible to isolate. As an example, consider the tautomeric forms of acetylacetone which are in rapid equilibrium with one another at room temperature:

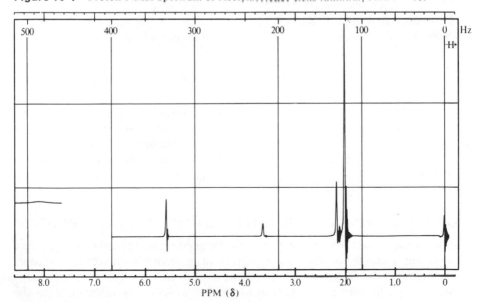

keto   enol

acetylacetone

The proton NMR spectrum of a sample of pure acetylacetone is shown in Figure 10-1. This spectrum is interpreted in the following way:

	group	δ
$-\overset{\overset{\displaystyle O}{\|\|}}{C}-CH_3$ (keto and enol)		2.05
$C=C-CH_3$ (enol)		2.2
$-CH_2-$ (keto)		3.65
$C=C-H$ (enol)		5.6
$-O-H$ (enol)		~ 15

Figure 10-1   Proton NMR Spectrum of Acetylacetone; CCl₄ Solution; Offset − 7δ.

The integral of this spectrum shows that the ratio of the area of the C=C—H resonance to the area of the $-CH_2-$ resonance is almost exactly 2 to 1. When one takes into account the fact that there is one C=C—H proton and two $-CH_2-$ protons, this 2 to 1 resonance area ratio indicates that the ratio of enol form to keto form is about 4 to 1.

DETERMINATION OF MOLECULAR WEIGHT

As indicated above, the integrated intensity of an absorption peak in the proton NMR spectrum depends only upon the molar concentration of the substance times the number of nuclei per molecule responsible for the peak. Thus the integrated intensity per nucleus per mole is the same for all substances in the sample. For this reason, when a known weight of a substance of known molecular weight (the standard—w_s/MW_s moles) is added to a sample containing a known weight of a substance of unknown molecular weight (the unknown—w/MW moles), the following equality must hold:

$$\frac{I_s/n_s}{w_s/MW_s} = \frac{I/n}{w/MW}$$

where I_s = integrated intensity of the peak of the standard
  n_s = number of nuclei responsible for the peak of the standard
  w_s = weight of standard added
 MW_s = molecular weight of the standard
  I = integrated intensity of the peak of the unknown
  n = number of nuclei responsible for the peak of the unknown
  w = weight of unknown used
 MW = molecular weight of the unknown substance
The molecular weight of the unknown substance may therefore be calculated. When the equality is solved for the molecular weight of the unknown, the result is

$$MW = \frac{I_s \cdot n \cdot w}{I \cdot n_s \cdot w_s} \cdot MW_s$$

For this method to be successful, a distinct resonance well separated from the rest of the spectrum is needed for both the unknown and the standard. For the unknown, a strong methyl singlet is excellent, though an isolated multiplet can be used. The standard is chosen so that its resonance will appear well separated from those of the unknown. Possible standards include iodoform (CHI_3) and 1,3,5-trinitrobenzene.

NMR SPECTROSCOPY OF NUCLEI OTHER THAN THE PROTON

Many nuclei other than protons have a magnetic moment and are therefore potentially suitable for analysis by magnetic resonance techniques. As Table 2-1 indicates, the frequency of rf radiation required for absorption of energy with a magnetic field at the nucleus of 14,092 gauss will be different from the

60 MHz needed for protons. Sometimes the same basic instrument can be set up for NMR spectroscopy of more than one kind of nucleus. but often a different instrument is used for each type of nucleus.

^{19}F NMR spectroscopy has been in use for almost as long as proton NMR spectroscopy since the isotopic abundance of ^{19}F is 100 percent, and the intrinsic sensitivity of the NMR method toward ^{19}F is almost as great as toward the proton. On the other hand, ^{13}C NMR spectroscopy has been employed only in recent years since ^{13}C occurs only in about 1 percent natural abundance (^{12}C, occurring in 99 percent natural abundance, is not magnetically active), and the intrinsic sensitivity toward ^{13}C is only 0.06 as great as toward the proton. Routine analysis of compounds containing ^{13}C at natural abundance had to await the development of highly sensitive NMR spectrometers and other techniques including time-averaging of many spectra (to average out random noise) and the far more efficient method of Fourier transform spectroscopy.

Since the relative abundance of ^{13}C is so low, it is improbable that a particular ^{13}C nucleus in a molecule will have a second ^{13}C nucleus as an immediate neighbor. Therefore splitting of a ^{13}C resonance by coupling to a neighboring ^{13}C nucleus is unlikely. If the protons in the molecule are spin-decoupled, as described above, the ^{13}C NMR spectrum of a substance will consist of a series of single peaks. In a favorable case, the number of structurally different carbon atoms in a molecule can be determined simply by counting the peaks in its proton-decoupled ^{13}C NMR spectrum. ^{13}C NMR spectroscopy promises to be of great use in the analysis of large, biochemically significant molecules since the spectra can be much simpler than the corresponding proton NMR spectra.

SHIFT REAGENTS

A class of compounds has been developed called "shift reagents." Upon addition to the NMR sample, a shift reagent causes chemical shift differences to be increased. The increase in chemical shift differences can make overlapping resonances move apart and can increase the $\Delta\delta/J$ ratio. For a spin system involving magnetic equivalence, an increase in the $\Delta\delta/J$ ratio can result in a more nearly first-order or $N + 1$ Rule spectrum. Figures 10-2 and 10-3 show proton NMR spectra of 2-methyl-3-butene-2-ol. The sample used for the two spectra was

2-methyl-3-butene-2-ol

the same except that a small amount of a shift reagent was added before the spectrum shown in Figure 10-3 was run. The addition of the shift reagent caused the overlapping lines of the vinyl resonance to move apart to reveal the expected three pairs of doublets (compare with Figures 4-11 and 7-6).

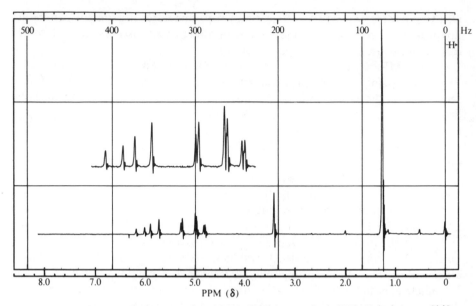

Figure 10-2 Proton NMR Spectrum of 2-Methyl-3-butene-2-ol; CCl₄ Solution; no Shift Reagent.

Figure 10-3 Proton NMR Spectrum of 2-Methyl-3-butene-2-ol; CCl₄ Solution; After Addition of tris-(2,2,6,6-tetramethylheptane-3,5-dionato)europium(III).

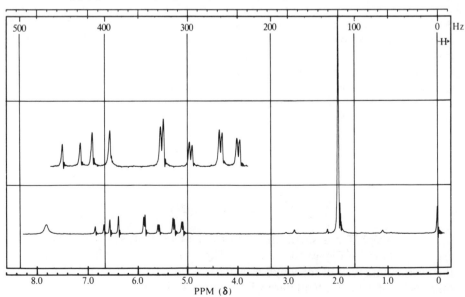

Figures 10-4 and 10-5 show proton NMR spectra of 2-methyl-2-butanol. The sample used for the two spectra was the same except that a small amount of

$$CH_3CH_2 \underset{\underset{\textstyle CH_3}{|}}{\overset{\overset{\textstyle OH}{|}}{C}} CH_3$$

2-methyl-2-butanol

a shift reagent was added before the second spectrum was run. As a result of the addition of the shift reagent, the distorted $N + 1$ Rule ethyl resonance of Figure 10-4 was changed to the more nearly first-order ethyl resonance of Figure 10-5 (compare with Figure 5-6).

In both examples, addition of the shift reagent causes all protons of the sample to be less shielded. The effect, however, is greater the closer the protons are to the site of coordination of the shift reagent (the oxygen atom). Therefore the position of the resonance of protons close to the oxygen will be changed more than the position of the resonance of protons distant from the oxygen, and the difference in chemical shift between such protons will be increased by addition of the shift reagent.

In both examples the resonance of the —OH proton was originally at $\delta = {\sim}3.4$. After addition of the shift reagent, it was moved in the first case to $\delta = 7.8$ (Figure 10-3), and in the second to $\delta > 8.3$ (Figure 10-5).

Figure 10-4 Proton NMR Spectrum of 2-Methyl-2-butanol; CCl_4 Solution; no Shift Reagent.

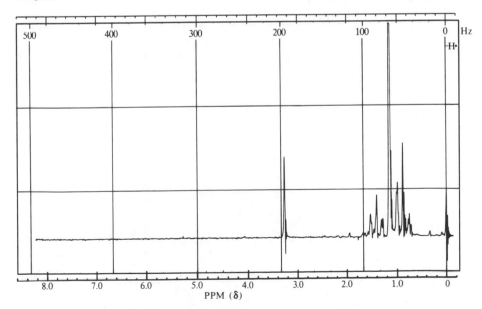

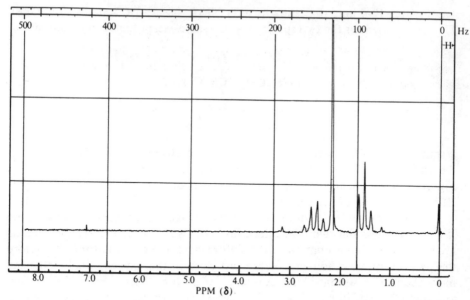

Figure 10-5   Proton NMR Spectrum of 2-Methyl-2-butanol; CCl₄ Solution; After Addition of tris-(2,2,6,6-tetramethylheptane-3,5-dionato)europium(III).

Figure 10-6   Proton NMR Spectrum of 60 mg. of an APC Tablet in 0.5 ml. CDCl₃.

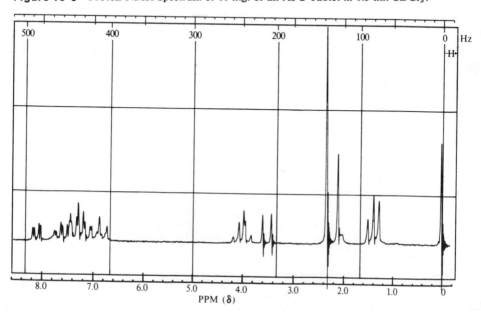

PROBLEM

Figures 10-6 and 10-7 present the proton NMR spectrum and integral of a solution of 60 mg. of an APC tablet in 0.5 ml. of $CDCl_3$. Estimate the relative amounts of aspirin, phenacetin, and caffein in the tablet. The spectra of these compounds are shown in Figures 7-15, 7-13, and 7-20.

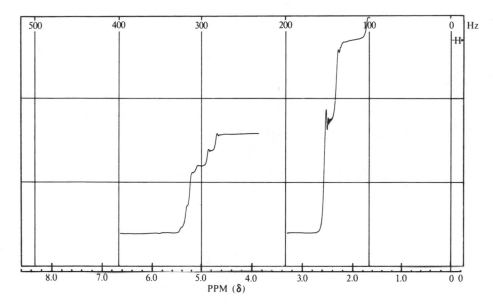

Left-hand trace: integral from $\delta = 5.3$ to $\delta = 2.8$.
Right-hand trace: integral from $\delta = 3.0$ to $\delta = 1.5$.

Figure 10-7   Integral of Spectrum Shown in Figure 10–6.

Index